WHAT I WISH
PEOPLE KNEW
ABOUT DEMENTIA

BY THE SAME AUTHORS

Somebody I Used to Know

WHAT I WISH
PEOPLE KNEW
ABOUT DEMENTIA

WENDY MITCHELL

with Anna Wharton

BLOOMSBURY PUBLISHING
LONDON · OXFORD · NEW YORK · NEW DELHI · SYDNEY

BLOOMSBURY PUBLISHING
Bloomsbury Publishing Plc
50 Bedford Square, London, WC1B 3DP, UK
29 Earlsfort Terrace, Dublin 2, Ireland

BLOOMSBURY, BLOOMSBURY PUBLISHING and the Diana logo are trademarks
of Bloomsbury Publishing Plc

First published in Great Britain 2022

A catalogue record for this book is available from the British Library

ISBN: HB: 978-1-5266-3448-1; TPB: 978-1-5266-4688-0;
EBOOK: 978-1-5266-3449-8; EPDF: 978-1-5266-4712-2

2 4 6 8 10 9 7 5 3

Typeset by Newgen KnowledgeWorks Pvt. Ltd., Chennai, India
Printed and bound in Great Britain by CPI Group (UK) Ltd, Croydon CR0 4YY

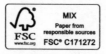

To find out more about our authors and books visit www.bloomsbury.com
and sign up for our newsletters

*Dedicated to my wonderful friend Sylvia, sadly
no longer here but never forgotten*

Contents

CONTENTS

INTRODUCTION

Here we are again. It is March 2021, and I am writing a second book after what has been a difficult year for all of us. I decided to write a follow-up to my bestselling memoir, *Somebody I Used to Know*, in the summer of 2020. The plan was for it to be published in 2022, and the first thing I said to my partner-in-writing, Anna Wharton, when I realised this was: 'I don't plan to be around then.'

Anna gently reminded me that I'd said this on publication of my first book in 2018, and yet here I still am.

As I write this, it has been almost seven years since my diagnosis of young-onset dementia and I still live alone, independently, without carers. What have I learned since that day in July 2014, when I sat in front of the neurologist and heard confirmation of those words that had been whispered to me in various letters and examinations in the lead-up to that date? Like many people, I knew nothing about dementia at the point of my diagnosis. All I did know were the snippets that we pick up, through the media, newspapers, television, perhaps a second-hand tale from a friend. I was frightened, of course, like most people. I was terrified of this progressive illness and its planned trajectory that would, slowly but surely, be revealed to me. I suddenly felt I had lost control of my own life, which is a very scary feeling – and also a very normal one.

So back to my question: what have I learned? Well, firstly, that I actually had much less to be afraid of than I thought. That yes, dementia is a bummer of a diagnosis but, like everything in life, it has a beginning, a middle and an end. Who knows where I am on my journey with this disease? What I see now, from this vantage point, is just a slice of the final sum total of my story with dementia. Is that really that dissimilar to how any of us live our lives? After all, the only certainty I have is the same as what everyone else has, which is actually just today.

But the reason I wanted to write this book is because I wanted to share with you just some of what I have learned about dementia – because I think it might surprise you, it might inspire you, it will definitely inform you, and, with any luck, it will help you to live the best life you are able to with the disease or support someone you know far better.

What has made the biggest difference to me are the people who I have met along the way. To be able to talk and share experiences with friends I have made who also live with dementia has made me feel more normal on days when the world seems a little fuzzy. To know that there are other people out there, struggling one day, thriving the next, but living all the same – not suffering (I hate that word) but living – makes a huge difference. And because they've made such a big difference to me, I wanted you to hear from them too, because my experience of dementia is *only* my experience. When you've met one person with dementia, you've simply met one person with dementia. We're as different as we all were before dementia. So it was important for me that this time round, you heard from others. Although you won't always read their names in the book, the voices that will share their experiences belong to the following people: Elaine, Eric, Eddy, Pat, Monica, Sue, Roland, Bob, Sue, Barbara, Colin, Brian, Janet, Paul, Delyse, Stewart, Gail, George, Dory and Agnes. All of these people are living with dementia in their fifties, sixties, seventies and eighties. Some have been diagnosed longer than me; some were diagnosed in the last couple of years.

When I was diagnosed, I had no idea where to start gathering information about what this new disease might look like for me. When you're diagnosed, you're suddenly meant to find out all this for yourself: no one contacts you to point you in the direction of support services or peer groups. You might not even be ready to attend any, maybe for months afterwards. But where, then, do you start? So often I hear: 'Well, we put out leaflets and posters.' But how do you know where to look for them, or what to look for?

I hope this book will at least give people a start. Imagine me while you are reading, gently taking you by the shoulders and steering you in the direction of some information I think you might find useful. I don't proclaim that this is an exhaustive list of answers to your questions, but it's a good place to begin.

When people think of dementia, they immediately associate it with memory. Few people realise, for example, just how it changes our relationships with our senses, our emotions, our communication. Few people understand the importance of a good environment – both inside and out – after a dementia diagnosis, and the small changes that can make a big difference. Unless you tell them, or talk about it, people will never know the difference dementia makes to your relationships – and how to make them work better. And if you don't know any of this at all, how can you be responsible for your attitude?

I hope I address all of these areas for you, whether you are someone living with dementia, someone supporting a person with the disease, a professional working in the field, or just a curious individual who believes that empathy and inclusivity is better for all of us – to you I extend an especially warm welcome. In these pages you'll find all the things that I wish people knew about dementia.

Wendy Mitchell
November 2021

SENSES

Like tiny bubbles rising to the surface in a pan of boiling water, memories can still surprise even those of us who have a disease that steals them. I thought of one the other day, of exactly that: my first home economics class, boiling a pan of water ready to receive an egg.

I had carried that egg to school tenderly, nestled inside a ball of wool. When I arrived at school, Mrs Marple, the home economics teacher, chastised me: 'Eggs belong in egg boxes,' she said.

We had learned quickly that she was a woman with a sharp tongue. We were all terrified of her, but this was the first year of secondary school and we felt very important carrying our ingredients into school each week in Tupperware.

'Today, we are going to learn how to boil an egg,' Mrs Marple told us during that first-ever lesson.

We listened to the instructions, taking care to write each stage neatly into our ruled exercise books. Placing the egg in a pan of water, making sure that it sunk to the bottom and didn't rise to the top, setting our timers and whipping the egg out of the boiling water at just the right time.

I had felt the breath of Mrs Marple on the back of my neck as she worked her way around the class observing each of us.

'Well done, Wendy,' she said, before moving on, leaving my classmate and I to share a relieved look.

Is that where I first attuned myself to such sensory pleasures? It's hard to say now. My mother wasn't a fan of cooking, or at least she didn't take the kind of pleasure in it that I did as I grew up. I can't remember what, if anything, she taught me in the kitchen. It was my father who I would find pottering around in there, sleeves rolled up to the elbow, hands white with flour, trying something with pastry. I did the same as a single mother, trying to be as inventive as I could to persuade tiny mouths to try some new delicacy. They were always more willing to try something that I made to fit their fingers – miniature pies and pasties, inside hidden more vegetables than I would ordinarily get away with feeding them. We watched *Masterchef* together as the girls tried to impersonate Loyd Grossman. Once a month we'd recreate the show, a chance for me to convince them to try new things as they graded me on the taster menu I had prepared for them: a tiny quiche topped with roast peppers or mackerel, a small risotto divided between three. The girls never needed much persuasion to eat the desserts, which would usually be the only course that got a ten out of ten.

It gets harder now to conjure up those memories – the smells of cookery, the consistency on the tongue of a cake baked to perfection. The ghosts of these scents perhaps still waft around my kitchen, though I wouldn't recognise them now.

ON HOW I EAT

Dementia changes our relationship with food, slowly eroding the enjoyment we once shared. I used to love the social opportunities that food afforded, a great vat of curry bubbling away on the stove, the air thick with spice, friends arriving, taking a seat around a table that I had adorned with a posy of flowers fresh from the garden. It's difficult to pinpoint a time when the social part of eating became difficult, when those conversations that criss-crossed the table became confusing to follow, when instead I would drop my napkin into my lap and sit back, listening without contributing. Or when the metallic clang of cutlery on a plate became too loud for my ears, leaving me feeling anxious and unsure.

Eating is such a sensory experience, not just in terms of taste and smell, but also touch, sound and sight. A black tablecloth left me confused about whether the table it covered was a giant sinkhole in the middle of the dining room, and once my eyes had adjusted or my brain had caught up and I realised it was indeed a tablecloth, I had no idea where the table started or ended underneath it.

Similarly, white plates became a problem. Serve a white plate of food to someone with dementia and fill it with pale mashed potatoes, or a flat, thin piece of fish, and they might not realise there is any food on the plate at all. Even our eyes aren't as hungry as they once were. We need contrast to distinguish whether there is food on the plate or not.

Once I understood that this was dementia at work, I decided to outwit it by buying bright yellow plates, figuring we don't generally eat many things that are bright yellow, scrambled eggs aside. But then even plates became problematic. My cutlery would chase the food around the plate until it fell unceremoniously off the edges, and once it wasn't there for me to see, it had simply never existed in the first place. I thought back to those times when I had sat my daughters in their high chairs and watched exactly the same thing happen. The solution to that had been fold-out tops that had a rim around them, harder for a baby to push food over the sides, and so I took my yellow plates to the charity shop, and instead bought bowls – big ones, pasta bowls. That way my food was less likely to evade me.

You will never realise until you have a complex disease inside your brain how complicated some of the everyday chores we take for granted really are. What appears to other people to be the simple act of using a knife and fork is actually a very complex process – a sawing action with one hand, while the other holds the food still. It reminds me of when young children learn to play the piano with two hands: at first it makes more sense for the brain to follow the other hand in unison – it is only with practice that each hand learns to play its individual keys. After my diagnosis I tried to eat the same way I always had, but suddenly the food escaped me, as if my hands weren't speaking to one another any more – a whole sausage would be pushed around a plate before being skewered by a fork and then held up for me to nibble pieces off. The act of cutting meat was difficult and laborious. It made me feel foolish that I could no longer eat without shame – but, I had to remind myself, what was the shame of having a disease inside my brain that was eating away at many of my abilities? Better to find a way to combat it. The answer came to me simply enough: to swap a knife for a spoon. The fork could do the cutting and the spoon could scoop it up afterwards.

Even when I had overcome that issue, meat remained a difficult food to swallow. It wasn't just the cutting up that it required, but the chewing too. When eating, it became impossible to remember how long I had been chewing, or how much longer I needed to chew. The result was, too many times, choking on food that I had not ground down enough before attempting to swallow. It's hard enough to concentrate on eating without the extra effort it takes to cut and chew. Meat had to go, and was replaced by fish.

Hot meals are difficult too. My dentist remarked recently on how many scald marks there are inside my mouth – I simply forget by the next mouthful that a hot potato has burned my mouth, and so I do it again.

It was difficult to know whether it was something neurological, or simply the new-found effort of eating that left me feeling neutral about food. Perhaps with nothing to replace the pleasure of a meal, or even preparing it, my brain simply switched off from the whole process. Or perhaps, as with many things, a circuit was lost inside my brain that meant I didn't feel hungry any more. Hungry *or* full, in fact. I eat now because I have to. I eat now for fuel. When I've mentioned just how little I eat on my blog, I have been inundated with offers of food parcels. Some less helpful people have even suggested that I was living with memory difficulties because I was starving my brain of vital nutrients. What those people don't know about dementia is that it doesn't just change *how* we eat, but what we eat.

ON WHAT I EAT
I used to love mushrooms with everything. I still think fondly of the simple pleasure that slicing them gave me,

little slivers of perfect toadstool shapes, the earth still clinging to them in places, as if they'd been delivered fresh from a forest floor. I'd cook them with butter and could never resist tasting one before assembling them on my plate. Even a simple supper of mushrooms on toast would sate my craving, and this I would repeat several times a week. Now I eat them and there is no pleasure in the texture or the taste. They taste of nothing. I may as well be chewing on cardboard.

Chillies were another thing I had with everything, a Spanish omelette being the favoured dish to slip them into – although really, for me, chillies went with everything. Whether they were emerald green or ruby red, my tongue was sharp and could distinguish flavours and colours. During my first pregnancy I had a craving for chillis on toast, and my daughter Sarah was born with a revulsion towards anything spicy until adulthood.

Each of these cravings I bade farewell to after my diagnosis, but one thing was non-negotiable and that was tea. It's impossible to conjure up the taste of mushrooms and chillies now and it's difficult to miss what you can't remember. But tea was different. Tea is more than a beverage; for me, it has always felt like a warm hug. Teacups became difficult to cope with, their tiny handles tricky and the attention that a cup and saucer demanded impossible to negotiate, and so I had a preferred mug, one that conducted the heat without burning me, keeping the tea warm as well as my hands. I liked to sit with each palm wrapped around it, savouring as much the ritual as the taste.

Evenings can be lonely events since my diagnosis, especially in winter when the sun sets while it's still afternoon

and darkness is difficult to navigate, but I never felt lonely
with a cup of tea for company. It sounds strange, but perhaps it's the emotional connection with tea that made its
memory linger longer with me – all those cuppas shared
with friends or loved ones, either in celebration or loss.
But then something started to change. Tea tasted funny,
different, and by that I meant different every day – one
day it even tasted of swede. I thought at first that it was
milk that was the problem. I experimented with just a
splash, and then none at all. I tried different varieties
rather than just my beloved Yorkshire Tea, but to no avail.
It seemed to me the cruellest trick: a disease that had
stolen so much from me had now taken such a simple
pleasure. I sat alone with a cup of hot water and lemon,
trying to recreate the friendship that tea had offered, but
it wasn't the same.

I have outwitted dementia on many other things. I have
accepted that my kitchen cupboards are ghosts of what
they once were. There are no longer cans and jars and
bottles jostling for space inside, cooks' ingredients desperate to be picked, pans stacked one on top of the other.
I said goodbye a long time ago to the gadgets I had for
everything. But nothing has replaced tea, and even though
I get no pleasure from it, I now just drink a very weak
Yorkshire Tea, simply to keep that connection.

Of course it makes sense that a complex brain disease affects not only the cognitive functions of eating and
drinking, but also the sensory experience and the motor
functions. I asked some of my friends how eating had
changed for them since being diagnosed with the disease.
Here are some of their replies:

'I used to cook because my husband can't cook, but we mostly eat ready meals now. I'm eating a lot less than I ever used to. I can never find the knives and forks. My husband tells me they've been in the same drawer for forty years, but I never know where they are.'

'I used to love eggs, but I don't eat them now, as I can't stand a fried egg or a boiled egg – I can't stand eggs now, and I can't eat meat any more.'

'I used to do all the cooking. I leave it to my husband now, but I feel guilty and I feel I should be doing it.'

'I don't cook. My wife does all the cooking, but I eat whatever is put in front of me.'

ON THE CHOICE OF FOOD

Decision-making can be a very complicated process when you have dementia. In my case, it means I often opt for the same thing to eat. Whenever I'm out and about, I buy a tuna sandwich. It saves the confusion that reigns in my brain if I'm given a list of choices or faced with counters of brightly packaged sandwiches with all sorts of fillings.

Dementia has made me an intuitive eater, too. In the same way that I more often rely on my gut instinct now to tell me whether I get a good vibe from a new person I meet, I listen more carefully now to the foods that my body demands. Most recently I experienced this with a craving for nuts and tomatoes and noticed, satisfied by whatever nutrient it wanted, that my body quietened down again. I get into the habit of preparing the same meals because it's easier. Often it can be a ready meal. In summer it might be a salad that is easy for me to make, given that it doesn't involve using the cooker – no chance of me wandering off and forgetting a pan on the boil. I had been eating that same salad and fish for months and months, but one day, well into autumn, I became very cold and just couldn't get warm. The cold was inside me, settled into my bones, and that evening I found myself unable to swallow my salad. The bowl of limp lettuce, tomato and cucumber stared back at me and I placed my fork down beside it. It was as if my body was refusing to eat it any longer. The following day I looked around the supermarket to see if I could find a ready meal that appealed to me. I came home with a lasagne and that night my body was happy again, and my bones were warm. By the following week, every shelf in my fridge had a lasagne on it.

I don't get sick of meals like others might, simply because I don't remember that it is the same one I had the night before. Food to me is fuel, nothing more complicated than that. Because I don't feel hungry, I set alarms on my iPad reminding me to eat. The only way I know whether I've eaten from one day to the next is if I see washing-up left on the drying rack.

Living alone makes it easy for me to have the autonomy to choose what I eat. There is no one to comment on the fact that I eat very little, or that I eat the same day after day. For those being supported at home, or in care homes, it may not be this simple. My experience is a common one; in fact, it is estimated that 50 per cent of people living with dementia will experience difficulty with eating, drinking or swallowing (dysphagia). This becomes more common as the disease progresses, but it can occur any time after diagnosis and yet it is not often talked about.

ON EATING IN CARE HOMES

Researcher Lindsey Collins recognises the way that eating and drinking changes after a diagnosis of dementia. She focused her PhD on understanding how this plays out in care homes. During her research, published in 2020, she looked at many different aspects of eating and drinking in care homes – whether that was the quality and choice of food on offer, the loss of identity in terms of being able to control what you eat or what time you eat, and how eating and drinking can still be an important part of socialising. Her conclusions made sad reading for me, particularly when it came to the choice of food on offer. It seemed that residents in care homes were often viewed as 'someone to be fed' rather than an individual with their own likes and dislikes. The truth is that these preferences don't disappear after a diagnosis with dementia.

'The eating and drinking experiences of people living in care homes were very different to their previous experiences of living in their own homes,' the report explained.

> The food quality and quantity had changed, as did the physical and social environment in which mealtimes and snacks took place. This resulted in experiences that were more negative than in the past and less focused on the individual's needs and preferences. For people living with dementia and dysphagia, the loss of identity and lack of recognition of individualised preferences was even more apparent … These individuals had each become merely someone to be fed, someone who was not afforded choice, someone who was given food and drinks that were often deemed unpalatable and lacking in variety.

When it comes to food, our likes and dislikes are so closely linked with our personality that I can understand why, if you take those preferences away from someone, you also strip them of their character a little.

I recognise that it would be impossible for care staff to take orders from each person individually. I also know that someone like me, who eats the same food day in, day out, sometimes for months, would be frowned upon – that I wouldn't be deemed as having a varied diet. But what's the alternative? If I were in a care home and was served up something I didn't like, or something that didn't taste nice, I would refuse to eat it. Then I would perhaps be labelled as a difficult patient, instead of anybody trying to get to the heart of why I couldn't eat it: could it be the taste? The plate it is presented on? Or the fact that the motor skills required to cut it up make it just too difficult to navigate?

Added to that, different variations of dementia affect people in different ways. For people who develop problems swallowing, eating might become so stressful that they would rather avoid it altogether. These people might also be seen as difficult for refusing food, when in fact a speech therapist might be able to help them, or a dietician might know what foods would be easier to swallow.

One thing that stood out in Lindsey Collins's research was the fact that mealtimes were still a vitally important time for residents to make connections, and this had a great impact on mental well-being. The report concluded: 'These positive experiences and connections were achieved through nourishing the person with the food and drink they enjoy, engaging the person in a meaningful way, seeing the person as the individual they are, and recognising the benefits which can be achieved through the simple daily act of eating and drinking.'

It makes perfect sense to me. You wouldn't enjoy a visit to a restaurant if you didn't like the food, so why would it be any different for those living with dementia?

There are things that care homes could do to help: they could remember that colour and contrast matter for people with dementia; swap cups and saucers for mugs; swap plates for bowls with rims that won't let food escape; offer a choice of no more than two or three things; cut up food to allow it to cool quicker, or remember not to serve it when it's piping hot; and keep disturbing noise and clatter to a minimum.

There are things that I have implemented to help eating become more enjoyable again. Sometimes a whole plate of food can feel like an enormous task to navigate. When my girls were little, I used to chop bits of fruit or vegetables up and place them in little bowls or ramekin dishes. This works well for me now. After dinner I usually put a few nuts in a ramekin dish, which is the perfect size for me: I can't have too many without realising and it enables me to pick them one after another, with no need to hurry.

If someone has enjoyed cooking in their life before dementia, there is nothing to stop them continuing now, with a little help. In the last days of my own home baking I found it difficult to follow a recipe or remember if I had already added an ingredient, but one of my friends manages to cook and her support worker keeps track of the ingredients she's added, or the length of time they have been cooking for.

There are still jobs that people living with dementia can have in the kitchen. Let us stir a pan, for instance, so that we feel part of the experience. People I know often talk about how they feel guilty for not helping, but we can still be useful – it just takes a bit of extra thinking to figure out how.

HammondCare in Australia has produced three cookbooks that address differing appetites after dementia, and speech and language therapists may be able to help those who have difficulty swallowing. It's also important to remember that some medications may impact the appetite, making it larger or smaller. They may even make the mouth drier, which makes eating less enjoyable. So check with your GP for more information about the side effects of certain medication.

Most importantly, for those caring for people with dementia, try not to take it personally if we refuse to eat the meal that you have prepared for us, or to judge us if we prefer to eat the same thing day in, day out. If someone is sitting with food in front of them untouched, it could be one of so many things, so please don't leap to any assumptions that they are being difficult, and try some troubleshooting instead.

ON BOILING AN EGG

I had almost given up totally on the idea of cooking again. There have been many kitchen disasters that have led me to this point: ruined food, burnt pans. In the end it was easier to turn off the cooker completely. But then, on one of my daily trundles around the village, something caught my eye. I pass the same house every day, sometimes pausing to take photographs of the two woolly sheep that stand in the field alongside it. As I do, I often hear the muted clucks of hens. But I had never noticed the little honesty box tucked just off the verge and the stack of freshly laid eggs beside it.

Could I remember how to boil an egg? I picked up one, perfectly shaped, and turned it around inside my palm.

At home, I stood once again in front of the cooker and a memory tugged at my sleeve: a pan bubbling away on each hob, steam filling the kitchen, scents of various home-cooked dishes mingling in the air above me. Instead now the room felt quiet and still.

My iPad was upstairs and there was no point trying to consult it; by the time I arrived upstairs to retrieve it, the question would have drifted away. And so I decided to start with the cooker. Who knew if it even worked any more? I turned the knob belonging to each burner. Nothing flickered or glowed orange with life, until the final one – the spark of a flame. I didn't know why it was that one in particular that I had been able to bring to life. Perhaps a muscle memory remained – had it once been my favourite? Who knew?

For boiling water I needed the kettle and decided it would be easier to fill the pan that way – lest I stand waiting for cold water to boil and get distracted and wander off. So I boiled the kettle, filled the pan, and gently placed the perfect little egg inside. I already knew I needed an alarm or two – I was aware that the moment I left the room, the egg and its pan of boiling water would cease to exist. But how long do you even boil an egg for? I thought again of the iPad upstairs, lying on my bed. I would have to guess, so I settled on eight minutes. I set the alarm beside the pan, the smallness of it belying the fact that it produces a big noise that I can barely stand. That, at least, would bring me rushing back to the cooker. I buttered two slices of bread to await the egg, then wandered into my sunroom, camera in hand and another alarm set on my phone, to snap pictures of animal visitors to my garden while I waited.

When an alarm sounded in my lap, I jumped, wondering what on earth it could be for – until I heard, seconds later, the shrill ring of the alarm in the kitchen. Of course, the boiling egg.

I had to think quickly what to do next – I realised cold water would cool the pan – so I filled it from the tap, waiting only a second before I fished the egg out. The tips of my fingers burned as I started to peel the shell, but a few moments later I cut it in half to reveal the jewel of the yellow yolk hidden inside. Sliced up on the buttered bread, it looked like a work of art. I swallowed it down with pride. I know this routine could all go wrong on another day – me distracted, for instance, by the tring of my iPad – but for now I was sated with the pleasure that dementia hadn't stolen this from me, my first 'home-cooked' meal in… well, I can't remember exactly how long.

ON SMELL

Like so many things in life, our sense of smell is something that we take for granted. And yet it is always there, cataloguing special moments in our minds. Years later the very same perfumes will come to us at random, steaming open the envelopes in our minds and spilling the contents. Or at least that's what my own sense of smell means to me. It is watching roses grow in the garden of our home as a child, fascinated by what nature could push from the soil and the heavy scent that would unfurl with their petals. It helped that, fully grown, these beautiful blooms were just the same height as me, perfect for dropping my nose into and inhaling deep lungfuls of their perfume. My mum loved roses and our garden at home was filled with all kinds of varieties. My favourites were the ruby-red Ena Harkness and the sunshine-yellow petals of the Peace rose, the edges pink as if tinted by the sun.

That memory, preserved by my nose, remained so strong that I tried to recreate it when I moved to the house I live in now. By then the name of my favoured roses had escaped me, and I knew my wobbly gait would mean I could no longer bend to bury my nose in the petals. Even so, I planted bushes of deep red flowers along my pathway, knowing that each time I brushed past them on the way to or from my front door the scent would rise to greet me. Each summer as the scent drifts up, I relive that childhood memory and something about it makes me feel safe and happy, reminding me of a different time.

It's not just flowers that have that effect on me. It's the smell of leather, the scent of my daughters' first T-bar shoes, which I keep in a box. These treasures are kept in the spare bedroom of my home, the place I call my memory room; it is a sanctuary where happy memories captured on film fill spaces on every wall. It's where I go when I need to sit and feel calm, surrounded by the people and places that have made me so happy. I've only to open the lid of that box containing the shoes and I'm there again, encouraging tiny feet into scuffed red shoes, out of the door and on the way to school. Money was tight as a single mum, but my own mother bought good leather shoes for both of my girls when I couldn't afford to. The smell of leather opens another envelope in my mind: a cream jacket my mum gave me the money to buy when I was fifteen. It was £20, which seemed a fortune in the late sixties, but it was so fashionable, short and fitted, soft and moulded to my body, and without a lining, its scent would linger on my clothes long after I'd hung it up. To this day, whenever I pass someone in the street and my nose captures that same rich, earthy and slightly sweet perfume, I am a teenager again.

It's not only the smells of my childhood that induce happy thoughts. There is a special place a few hours from home, alongside my own piece of paradise that is Derwentwater in Keswick. Follow the path clockwise around the lake and, just after the centenary stone, you will come across a pine copse. One foot inside and a sharp, sweet, slightly citrusy scent embraces you. It is enough for me in those moments to just stand still and breathe in the fresh smell, the silence interrupted only by the crunch of pine needles under my feet. I don't need to be in my beloved Lake District to have that same feeling of peace – wherever I am, a whiff of pine transports me in seconds to that same happy place.

Our olfactory system is a treasure trove of memories and emotions for all of us. Olfaction is the only one of the senses that does not traverse the thalamus, the usual relay station for our sensory signals. Instead, it speeds directly through the hippocampus, an important area for memory, and the amygdala, which has a strong connection to emotions. For this reason, there have been studies on how effective memory recall is in people living with mild dementia, using their sense of smell as a prompt. A 2018 Japanese study found that as a cue for recollection in the elderly population, retrieving a memory through olfactory stimulus can be more effective than through conversation alone, and that this could improve mental health more generally. The report said: 'It is easier for elderly people to recall past memories and emotions during intervention when practising reminiscence using olfactory stimuli compared with when practising reminiscence using conversation. Such intervention results in emotional stability and, consequently, may affect the tendency to decrease depression during intervention in the short term.' No wonder I love my rose-lined pathway so much.

Another 2019 French study found that when using odour to enhance recall, people living with Alzheimer's were able to retrieve a higher number and more specific recent memories, as well as those relating to their childhoods and adult lives.

'The decline of autobiographical memory in Alzheimer's disease has been associated with negative effects on identity and the sense of self in patients,' researchers concluded. 'Our study demonstrates how the decline of autobiographical memory in Alzheimer's disease can be, to some extent, alleviated by odour exposure … In our view, olfactory stimulation should be implemented in clinical rehabilitation programs aimed at improving autobiographical retrieval.'

When stimulated, our sense of smell can be a useful resource in alleviating the decline of autobiographical memory. A 2020 French study set out to discover which part of 'ourselves' it could prove useful in rediscovering.

The findings showed that those with dementia who were asked to recall autobiographical details about themselves using various pleasant odours tended to focus more on psychological statements, for example what kind of a person they were (caring, happy, friendly, lucky, etc.), rather than what they did for a living, or descriptions of their physical self.

'While previous studies have shown the beneficial effect of odour exposure on the retrieval of autobiographical memories in Alzheimer's disease, this study is the first to demonstrate that odour might be an effective cue to enhance access to self-concept in Alzheimer's disease patients,' researchers concluded.

The loss of self has been linked to a decline in the health of people living with dementia, so understanding ways in which we can hang on to our memories and our stories may prove helpful in understanding the disease and preserving the person. There has also been research into whether a loss of sense of smell can be an early indicator of Alzheimer's, although the jury is still out on that one. One study found that among patients who have a genetic risk of developing Alzheimer's, risk of the disease was five times higher in those who had lost their sense of smell.

ON OLFACTORY HALLUCINATIONS

Unfortunately, our sense of smell doesn't always grant us pleasant memories. Many people with dementia report olfactory hallucinations, and almost always they are not scents you would prefer to have in your nose.

This has happened to me many times. On one occasion, watching television, I could suddenly smell that distinctive whiff of fire. I darted about the house searching for flames and even went outside looking for a fire, but there was nothing. Time has taught me to understand that it's unlikely that these smells really do exist. But when it happens, it feels as real to me as sticking my nose in that rose. According to research, olfactory hallucinations tend to last for the same period of time as aural or visual ones – that is, between a few seconds and a minute. A quick survey of my friends revealed that these hallucinations are very common:

'I often smell wood burning. I don't find it offensive, as it's quite a nice smell to me. I know of other folk who experience nasty smells, though.'

'I've never had a cat, but I spent months convinced that a cat was sneaking into my home and using it to pee. I lifted my front door tiles and relaid them to try and rid me of the smell. Now I burn essential oils like lavender.'

'My husband, who has dementia, kept smelling petrol. I was checking all his clothes in case he had spilt some on him in the garage. It was a long time before I realised they were hallucinations.'

'I smell burning bonfires. It's awful; it happens any time, anywhere. I hate it. It even makes my nose sting.'

'I smell burning, rotting cabbage, dirty, stale mops and drains – I wish I smelled flowers.'

It's easy to see why these hallucinations might be distressing to people who experience them without understanding that they can be a normal part of the disease. It's important, as with all these tricks of the brain, that those supporting people living with dementia understand this too. If we tell you we can smell something, in that moment it smells completely real to us. Knowing these things means a better relationship with the disease for everyone.

A friend of mine, Dr Jennifer Bute, is an ex-GP who was diagnosed with dementia in 2009. After she retired, she went on to write a book about her experience of the disease, *Dementia from the Inside: A Doctor's Personal Journey of Hope*. I spoke to her about her experiences of olfactory hallucinations, and she said:

'Some people believe dementia creates hallucinations from nowhere, but it does not do this. Dementia isn't "making up" the hallucination, it just "releases" stored memories from the past, and unfortunately usually the unpleasant ones.

'I have hallucinations of dreadful smells, but I worked in the slums of Calcutta and New Delhi in India and the "memories" of these awful smells are fixed in my mind because of the intense feelings created by them.

'I have frequent olfactory hallucinations of burning. I have ended up with fire engines at my home before. I certainly have memories of fires from my past, so perhaps that is these memories resurfacing. The boarding school I attended was burned down because one pupil had a toaster under their bed and forgot to turn it off.

'So what releases these hallucinations? For me, I've noticed that it is if I am overtired, or have forgotten my medication, or occasionally if I am under a lot of pressure from people, or places I need to go.'

Understanding these hallucinations and, like Jennifer, noting particular patterns as to when they occur, might give us clues to help lessen their frequency – particularly if they are unpleasant to experience. The rule that helps me cope with hallucinations, be they visual, aural or olfactory, is my thirty-minute one. I tell myself that if I see something that seems unusual, distressing or doesn't seem right, I should leave it for thirty minutes, go away and do something else. If I return and it's still there, it's not a hallucination. Of course, this has never happened.

I know some of my friends keep a scent of something nice nearby so that if they experience a hallucination, they can plunge their nose into something that smells more pleasant. The problem is, it can be difficult to remember to keep that something alongside you.

ON HEARING

Dementia distorts your reality on a daily basis. That bang you heard outside that sent a chill all the way up your spine? It didn't exist. A firecracker, the sound of a mad gunman on the loose? These aural hallucinations leave you pinned to your armchair, heart racing, too terrified to look outside. The sounds that dementia conjures up in my brain are as real to me as the pages of this book you are reading now. Yet one brave look out the window proves there is no one rampaging the street with a sawn-off shotgun. That light *rat-a-tat-tat* at the front door? There is never anyone on your doorstep when you open it.

All of these are tricks of a diseased brain, but ones that no one warns you about. I remember how, back in the very early days of my dementia, this new disease changed the landscape of the beloved city of York, where I lived. I loved my riverside apartment; it was, I had decided, my forever home. Yet suddenly, it was as if the city had turned up the sound dial. Every step outside of my home was more and more overwhelming. Now hazards awaited me on every street corner: the piercing ring of ambulances that stopped me in my tracks, clutching at my head to still the pain; the growl of car engines as they waited for lights to change; a gabble of voices that could render the Shambles disorientating and frightening. It was as if my city and I had become strangers to one another overnight. Yet no professional had warned me this was a symptom of the disease inside my head. For me, this change in my hearing was puzzling – I had never had any problems before. Dementia was an illness that affected the memory, so there must be something else wrong with me, I supposed. I wasn't then used to the many ways in which dementia can render our worlds unfamiliar, some things taking hold slowly, and others almost overnight.

Had a professional warned me that I might experience these sensory changes, perhaps anxiety would not have accompanied me outside with each footstep. Perhaps I wouldn't have worried that another part of me was failing. Instead, my light-bulb moment came when one of my friends, Agnes Houston, happened to mention in passing that her own sensitivity to noise had developed since she had been diagnosed with dementia. Agnes had spoken to others like me who had noticed changes to their vision, hearing, taste and smell, and had realised that no doctor had warned any of us about this. Worse still, many so-called experts didn't even know that these sensory changes were a part of the disease. So Agnes embarked on her own research, writing a book alongside Julie Christie, *Talking Sense: Living with Sensory Changes and Dementia*, which explores the impact of dementia on the senses. I would recommend it to anyone living with the disease.

I asked some of my other friends what their experience had been of aural hallucinations:

'Sometimes I say to my wife: "Did you shout?" and she says: "No." And I say: "Well, somebody shouted, I heard it."'

'I'm always hearing my husband speak, but he says he hasn't said anything.'

'Sometimes when I'm walking to the shops, I'll stop and say: "You walk in front because I walk too slowly." When I turn around, there's nobody there, but you swear you've heard somebody.'

It turned out there was a name for the sensitivity to sound that I experienced: hyperacusis. This is a condition that affects how you perceive sounds. You can experience a heightened sensitivity to particular tones that aren't a problem for other people, which means that loud noises that startle you, like fireworks, or even loud everyday noises like the shrill ring of a telephone, can feel uncomfortable or painful. But it was five long years after my diagnosis with dementia that I would hear that word for the first time. The doctor I saw after a year on the waiting list was very open to listening, admitting that he didn't know anything about dementia and hearing. At least he admitted

it. He tested my hearing and it transpired that I wasn't
hearing high pitches (which can be a normal part of ageing)
but I reached the point at which it becomes uncomfortable
very quickly. With low pitches, I have a larger range of
hearing, but it's still a lot smaller than it might be in others
before it becomes uncomfortable.

Despite the diagnosis, there wasn't anything that particular hospital department could do to help me because
I'd been referred to the wrong one. Handed around, as
is often the case with the NHS, I took my place on yet
another waiting list. But that appointment would prove
life-changing. Rebecca Dunn is a clinical physiolo-
gist specialising in audiology at Hull and East Yorkshire
Hospitals NHS Trust. I liked her immediately: she took
the time to explain exactly what was going on inside my
head and showed me graphs of my hearing range. The ideal
is a straight line, but mine veered wildly across the page.
She told me how there is a gate between the ears and the
brain. The gate works by opening and closing – particularly when we hear a loud noise that would equate to a
sensory overload. The problem with my gate, and the gate
of anyone who lives with hyperacusis, is that it is perman-
ently open, so to me, a loud noise feels like a raging bull
crashing through my head.

'Earplugs wouldn't work,' she told me, 'because they
wouldn't close the gate.'

It suddenly made sense to me then why my own 'home
remedies', the earplugs I'd bought myself to dull the world,
hadn't worked. They'd simply quietened sounds I needed
to hear, like a car approaching, so could have actually been
quite dangerous. What Rebecca suggested were hearing

aids that would block off the range of noises that I found particularly uncomfortable. They changed my whole outside life. Finally I could stand on a train platform and not flinch and clutch at my head when a train came into the station. I could walk the streets on shopping trips without jumping back into people as a motorbike passed me, or cower as an ambulance, its siren blaring, raced by.

Rebecca told me that the key to understanding how hearing is affected for those living with dementia lies in looking at the patient more holistically. I went back to speak to her about what can be done to help people living with the disease:

'I would say that the dementia patients I see who may have hearing issues are further along than they should be,' she explained. 'It's always the basics that concern the carers, and we need to get there earlier in terms of establishing sensory changes in those living with dementia. Ideally, this would mean that all dementia patients are hearing-screened on diagnosis, because if you can help patients before the hearing and their environment becomes more threatening or anxiety-provoking, then you stand a greater chance of reducing something like hyperacusis. But at present, we don't have a budget to test all dementia patients. I know dementia staff are keen to join our different areas, but there needs to be a better understanding of how the two are affected.

'I come at a person from a neurophysiological background, so I approach my clinic from the premise that the patient needs to understand the problem they're experiencing in relation to their own personal circumstances. Once they understand this, they have more agency and are able to make informed decisions about what they would like to do, and if they can improve their situation. Hyperacusis is a natural reaction to a challenging environment where an animal is unsure of its safety – the more triggers they have to feel unsafe, be they historical or current, the more likely it is that they will have a problem. So if hyperacusis in dementia patients is caused predominantly because they don't feel safe in their environment, then we can work to make that environment feel safer, and place safety nets there so that the person is less stressed and therefore won't get an overload of sensory information, because their perceived danger is reduced.'

I'm not stressed when I'm in the street; I do feel safe and I forget about sirens until they are upon me. But I appreciate where she is coming from: we need to look at ways to make every environment more dementia-friendly, and this for me meant programming the hearing aids to make my environment better.

Rebecca took the time to try to understand dementia and all the challenges that it brings. I was amazed when she said that I've probably not heard 'S' and 'T' sounds in words, which explained why I couldn't always follow conversations. With the hearing aid set correctly, they returned. As she pointed out, these subtle differences are the same as going to an optician and them putting different lenses in front of your eyes to make letters sharper.

As with anything concerning dementia, when it comes to sensory changes, it's about the individual and not the disease itself. But when it comes to making environments more dementia-friendly, there are still things that hospitals and other places of care can do to help people visiting.

For those dealing with hyperacusis, it would be helpful for the audiology department to be situated somewhere away from the main hub of the hospital when sounds like clanging metal and slamming doors can be so disorientating. Yes, we must listen to doctors – they can impart useful information that will help us better cope with our new worlds – but they need to listen to us too.

ON VISION

It's not often that you hear people talking about how vision is affected by dementia. It's not our eyes that are the problem, but the way the brain interprets the messages it receives from them. If I am at the top of a staircase, for example, it is difficult to decipher if it is an escalator that will move when I step onto it, or a slide that I'll slip down like a child in a playground. If the steps are covered in the same carpet or surfacing, I can't see each individual step, so I don't know where to put my feet. The best kind of treads are those where the edges are clearly marked, particularly in yellow, as is often the case with outdoor staircases. I decided this is why I so often fall up and down my stairs at home, as they are carpeted with no clear edge. Now I have two stair banisters, one on each side, to hold on to to make it less likely.

Patterned carpets are completely disorientating because all the shapes just seem to come alive, moving around in front of my eyes. It can be very disconcerting to be asked to walk across a carpet that looks as though it's covered with wriggling creatures, and because many of us with dementia have a wobbly gait, we tend to spend a lot of time looking at the floor to make sure we don't fall over.

A shiny marble floor just looks like a swimming pool. Imagine trying to walk on water. Black mats by doors look like gaping great sinkholes in the ground. Black is generally a very bad colour for some of us. Now if I see someone dressed in black, it looks like their head is floating in thin air. A mounted flat-screen TV just looks like a huge hole in the wall. Now, when I visited my beloved B & B in Keswick, the owner, Catherine, puts a red pillowcase over the TV in my room before I even arrive.

It is tone and contrast that are difficult for our brains to distinguish, which means a carpet the same colour as the walls is just impossible to navigate. The easiest way to find out if a room or an area is dementia-friendly is to take a black-and-white photograph. If the contrast between shades of black, white and grey is obvious, then it should be OK. Colour, of course, is a personal choice, but it's always the contrast that matters. For example, black writing on a yellow background works well, or the NHS blue colour on a white background is clear. I always used to wear black, but now I like bright colours because they're easier to find – now my navy coat is hardly worn in favour of my yellow one.

Here's what some of my friends had to say about how their vision has changed:

'I have a problem looking for things. I can't always visualise what things look like to find them. So if I'm looking for my phone, I can't picture what my phone looks like. It's the same with my glasses, especially if my glasses are in their case. In my mind, the shape of what I'm looking for has disappeared.'

'Looking for something in a handbag is difficult because it's black inside, so I like coloured things, like I have yellow tape around my glasses case so it looks different, and a red phone. Black is difficult for finding things.'

Dementia can be cruel in so many ways, yet every so often it hands us a gift in a most unexpected form. It was a bright day in the garden, and the sun was starting its descent, streaking long shadows of the fence across the lawn. I was pottering inside, shuffling from one room to another with a cup of tea in hand, trying to decide where to sit. Suddenly, through the glass of the double doors, something caught my eye. It took a while for the silhouette to make a recognisable figure, but it was then that I saw the unmistakable shape of him: a man, standing in the middle of my lawn – my father.

By then he must have been dead twenty years; should I have been frightened to see him in all his incredible, yet very ordinary detail? He was wearing his familiar baggy green cardigan, his happy, casual clothes that he wore to potter in his own garden shed, and on his face was the same relaxed smile. A tip of mine for visual hallucinations is to take a photograph on your phone or iPad of what you think you can see, and if it's in the picture, it's most likely there in real life. But in that moment, I did not want to break the spell. He stood, just looking at me, his hands hanging by his side, even the yellow of his nicotine-stained fingers visible from this distance. His hair was styled with Brylcreem, as it always was, black and shiny, the last of the sun reflected back from the black quiff that never went grey. I was reminded, as we stood looking back at one another, of the times I would climb into his lap as a small child and he would pay me a penny per grey hair that I could find and pull from his scalp. The memory of that moment returned me to the warmth of his touch, the sweet sugary scent of his Brylcreem and its bright red pot.

I don't know how long we stood looking at each other. It could have been minutes or hours – dementia has a funny relationship with time. The logical part of my brain knew that what I was seeing what was not real. I know the disease has a habit of playing tricks on my brain, and normally I would use my thirty-minute rule – walking away and returning half an hour later to know for sure whether what I saw was still there. But this time I simply stopped and stared, determined to enjoy this gift that dementia had granted me, because they are so few and far between. I felt not fear but an emotional pull to stay and spend some time in the company of my dear old dad again.

I play this cat-and-mouse game with dementia on a daily basis, and all too often it beats me. But that day, I knew that dementia had got it wrong. Instead of frightening me, it had blessed me with a visit from someone long gone and much missed. I knew Dad was content by the clothes he was wearing, and so was I, on that sunny afternoon, my cup of tea cooling in my hand. I looked down at it, and when I looked up again, he was gone.

ON DREAMS
Do dreams count as hallucinations? If our brains can run riot in the day, then why not at night? My dreams have

definitely changed post my dementia diagnosis. Sleep now is a visitor who drops in infrequently. Most nights are spent lying in bed, my eyelids closed, my eyeballs staring into the nothingness behind them. At first I would find this night-time routine exhausting, but now I have given in to it. I simply lie there, allowing my body to relax, waiting for the morning, grateful for any few minutes that I drift off, in and out of the blackness of the night.

It is said that people regress to a different era in the latter stages of this disease, that the mind somehow chooses a shelf of a former life in the great bookcase that makes up our story. I no longer dream of the present, only the past. It's as though my dreams have regressed before my brain has, and are opening a window to the reality that I may be immersed in during the later stages of dementia. Perhaps my dreams return me there because, for a time, it was a happy period in my life. My daughters are always young, usually around six and three. Sarah is often doing an adult job like working in an NHS call centre – she sits, all three feet of her, at a giant desk in an oversized office chair, her feet dangling mid-air, unable to quite reach the floor. Gemma is still a tiny child and I am a young mum – our roles reversed just for that moment in time, when once again it is me holding their hands. In my dreams I rarely have dementia, which should be comforting, until I wake and find it keeping me company on the pillow.

Why do I think this is a sign of things to come? Because it is the place my subconscious so naturally leads me back to. I was happy then, after all, before the split with my husband. I felt safe in those days, no worries but the care of my two growing girls, their complete and utter reliance on me giving me a purpose I perhaps feel is lacking now. Those moments our minds settle on feel as real to us as the day-to-day you are living, yet they can be frustrating for and misunderstood by those around us. Take, for example, an anecdote I heard of a woman in a care home who would repeatedly tap her table. So relentless was this tapping that the staff called her family over from Australia to find her a new home because her behaviours were so disruptive to carers and residents. It was only when her family revealed what she had done in her life pre-dementia that her habit made sense – she was a codebreaker at Bletchley Park during the war, and the constant tap-tapping was how she used to send codes. Dementia had just delivered her back to that time in her life.

But more and more now, day and night, dreams and reality are becoming harder to separate and decipher. I woke up the other morning, heart thumping with confusion, and I immediately reached for my iPad to write down what had happened while I still remembered all the details. I'd gone for a walk, which takes me down a footpath alongside the bypass, only I'd got into a pickle with the turning and found myself heading down the embankment onto the bypass. I knew something wasn't right – I remember thinking that the drop is not usually that steep – but once I'd started, momentum just took me to the bottom. I looked this way and that and felt so vividly the speed of the cars rushing past me, so close they made me catch my breath. The noise was unbelievable. Looking back, I knew I'd never be able to climb back up the verge and so I had no choice but to walk. I was sure – so sure – I would come to an exit, a slip road or a roundabout. But then a car coming towards me began to slow down, and I saw the familiar blue flash of the lights on top. It was the police.

I told them how I'd got confused and had veered from my normal route. They wanted to take me back to the spot to see the gap that had made me go wrong, but I felt so guilty, so silly for wasting their time, knowing they'd have to do a massive detour to drive me back there. They were kind and persuasive, explaining how much further I would need to walk to find an exit. I suddenly looked at their uniforms and wondered if they really were the police, but then, what choice did I have but to go with them?

We went on the long detour, them keeping me in conversation, me reluctant to reveal my dementia, until finally we arrived back to the site of my misdemeanour. They could see the damage to the barrier that had allowed me through, and I showed them the footpath a few yards away that I had strayed from. Suddenly a man appeared, saying hello to me by name. Apparently he was from the village and knew me well. He took one of the policemen aside and as they were chatting I heard him say quite clearly: 'She has dementia; she can get confused sometimes.' I stood there, trapped, guilty as charged.

He waved goodbye after a while and the policemen said they'd better take me home. I hadn't been able to go for my trundle and I protested, but they said: 'We'd feel better if we took you home today – there's always time for another walk tomorrow.'

I felt the panic then. I didn't want them to know I lived alone. I wondered what they would do – report me to the authorities? Raise the alarm with social services? I sat in the back of the police car, mouth dry, head spinning. As we crossed the traffic lights to the village, they asked me my address and somehow I had the forethought to tell them my daughter Gemma's address instead, just hoping she and her husband Stuart would be there.

As we pulled up outside, an anxious Stuart appeared at the door, followed by Gemma.

'I got in a pickle on my trundle and the police brought me home,' I told them before they could say anything.

Thankfully the police didn't ask any questions and left me there and went on their way, hopefully fighting crime and forgetting all about me.

That's when I opened my eyes and I couldn't figure out whether all that had really happened. I looked around my bedroom; I was in my own bed. But the images and the feelings were so real, and my heart still thumped, my head was still whirling. I lay there trying to work out if it was what had happened yesterday. I wanted to text Gemma, but then didn't want to worry her if it was all a figment of my subconscious.

Reality or a dream? I'm still not sure…

ON TOUCH

As babies, we crave the touch and reassurance of our caregivers. As mothers, we long for the feel of our baby's skin next to our own. I still remember the hours spent feeding my own daughters, their hands reaching up to grasp at mine – tiny fingers wrapping carefully around my own. In those early days, whether human or animal, touch is so important, an instant communication between mother and young. Perhaps, with dementia, we return to our animal instincts, intuitive contact taking on a greater importance to make us feel safe.

As my daughters grew, so did their confidence. Those hands that once clutched tight to mine on the way to and from school now wanted to strike out on their own. There were still night-time hugs or cuddles when the day had got too much for them, or if there was something to celebrate. The truth is that we never grow too old to forget the importance of human touch. Except for the fact that, apart from with my daughters, I was never a very tactile person. Dementia changed that: suddenly I found myself wanting to hug everyone that I met, or at least the people who I knew by instinct that I liked. I see people as kind or not kind, and for those who show kindness, in return I wanted to hug them to show my gratitude. Their kindness means much more than they can imagine. I suddenly found myself hanging on to my daughters for longer and harder. Was it lost inhibitions that were to blame? A new neediness I hadn't been brave enough to admit to? Or perhaps a hug represents an inner emotional reserve: maybe touch cuts through moments when words grow complicated or hard to find, instantly communicating that someone cares.

It could also be that living alone plays a part in my new reliance on touch. For me there is no arm of comfort when I need it. Is it any wonder that sometimes I want to hold on to my daughters and not let them go? I have become used to many role reversals in my journey with dementia – it is now my daughters who want to know where I am, or what time I'm expected home – and it's now me who needs their touch for safety, reassurance, to know that I am not alone.

Touch remains more vital to all of us than we are perhaps willing to admit. Maybe we see it as some kind of weakness to admit that we need to feel another's hand on our own. Perhaps the reserved pre-dementia me, who'd been let down in life by men, didn't want to feel touch again; I felt a hug was for a deeper relationship that I wanted to avoid. That fear of being hurt again kept me at a distance from anyone. But when dementia came along, that fear vanished. It was suddenly insignificant compared to this new challenge I had to face.

Take human touch away from those living with dementia and we miss it dreadfully – even if we don't want to admit it. A 2011 Australian study found that a ten-minute foot massage once a day changed the behaviour of people living with dementia in long-term care. Residents of a care home in Brisbane were described as having 'agitated behaviour', which according to the study included aggression, wandering or repetitive questioning. (I hate the phrase 'agitated behaviour': it always strikes me that the behavioural 'problems' might be less to do with the person living with dementia themselves and more to do with their need to be understood by their caregivers. It's just a bugbear of mine.)

What researchers discovered was that a ten-minute foot massage by trained professionals reduced this 'agitated behaviour' dramatically – even for two weeks after the massages stopped. This was put down to the fact that 'massage fosters a sense of meaningful communication even when language skills have declined'. These 'behaviours' are often treated with medication that can have side effects, or worse still, with physical restraints. With a massage, on the other hand, there are only benefits: the eye contact with the person who is doing it, perhaps a little conversation, the focus on the sensation applied to the skin.

This research is useful for caregivers who are supporting people living alone with dementia. My daughter Sarah, a nurse, uses hand massage at work to relax patients. It is a little something that anyone caring for a person living with dementia could do. It's not unusual for carers to feel disconnected from the person they are supporting, unsure of how to demonstrate the bond between them, but a hand massage is a way of showing this. It says something more meaningful than words, perhaps: it shows that someone is taking their time to relax with you, and that the recipient is worthy of that time. It actually speaks a thousand words.

During my fogs, if I feel someone's hand reaching for mine, guiding me if I am confused, disorientated, lost or out of my depth in a new place or among new people, it can be such a relief. When we are unstable physically, we need that hand to lean on or to lead us, or just to comfort us with the knowledge that someone is there, that we can take our time and that things will be OK. When the fog is lingering and life is less clear, a hand on ours is a way of drawing our attention, of gently leading us back to the moment and calming the storm. That touch says 'I'm here'. There is no need for words.

My daughter Gemma started cutting my hair for me back in 2020. She was tentative at first, worried about making a mistake, despite the fact I told her that I wasn't worried what I looked like. But it wasn't just the haircut – it was the time we spent together. The closeness, the chatter and kind, caring touch made us both feel good.

Three weeks after my first trim, I went back for a tidy-up. Gemma was much more confident this time, the laughter between us got louder, and I only realised her concentration had slipped when the buzz of the clippers she was using sounded odd. I looked up in time to catch the horror on her face.

'I bet that was a number-two clipper, not a number seven,' I said.

'Could well be,' she said.

We fell about laughing. At least hair grows back.

RELATIONSHIPS

I can still see Gemma and Sarah, cross-legged on the floor as children, attempting to learn how to tie their shoelaces. They must have each been about five or six when they first tried, their tiny fingers tying nothing but themselves in knots trying to complete what must have seemed like such an impossible task. Up until that point I had bought them shoes with buckles that were easy to slip their feet into, two quick clips and we were out the door: to the park, the playground, the shops – adventures coming thick and fast back then. But then came time for laces, their pleas for the same shoes as their friends – the same friends who had already mastered the art of weaving those laces between metal eyelets. How grown-up that skill must have felt to my girls; no wonder they were so determined to crack it. And so we practised, over and over and over again. I never hurried them out the door, never flustered those young minds as they sat there, determined to thread and weave, pinching lace between forefinger and thumb and making bows.

I could picture myself as a small child in those moments too, sitting on the red patterned Axminster carpet in front of an open fire. The shame of my laces having come undone at school, having to ask the teacher for help and the cruel jibes of the boys still burned at my cheeks. Now

I witnessed the same determination to learn on the faces of my girls.

I bought them a brightly coloured cardboard cut-out shoe, with holes and lace threaded through, and how many hours we must have sat together practising the art of tying them before finally one of them stood up, face beaming, eyes bright, and wandered across the living room to show me what they had finally achieved.

After that, the simplicity of such an everyday task must have felt so obvious to them. But wasn't that my role as their mother? To help my daughters find a way through each seemingly dead end they came across in life; to equip them with the skills necessary to overcome each task on their way to independence. We bring our children into the world to leave us. We nurture their talent, achievements and skills to a point where they can fly the nest. We encourage them to try new things and soothe them when it fails the first time, providing them with sanctuary for sometimes nothing other than their ego. And then we push them back out into the world. Or at least I did.

Nowhere on that roadmap of their lives was there anything that indicated that our roles would be reversed, that one day they would be looking after me – or even helping me tie my own shoelaces. But life has a funny way of coming full circle.

I'd had the same walking shoes for twenty years. Once laced, they saw me up and down the Three Peaks as well as miles and miles of other terrain and Lakeland walks. I hadn't been expecting the day when I stared down and had no idea how to tie them: the laces hung at the sides of each shoe, as scrambled to my brain as a messy ball of wool. I felt helpless, hopeless, and it was left to Sarah to kneel down in front of me to tie them – just as I had once done for her. This wasn't how I imagined it would be or how I wanted it to be. In that one small gesture, it felt that so much had changed and I wasn't willing to accept it. I wasn't ready for my daughters to be carers. Not now, not ever. Instead, I had to find another way.

The answer, when it came, was simple enough: no-tie shoelaces. Sarah replaced my old ones for me, and with one tug of both hands, my old faithful shoes were done up as tight as before. Another problem was thwarted – the next might not be so easy – but my independence was sustained for another day.

ON CARING

Don't be fooled into thinking that a diagnosis of dementia is just for one person. Yes, the disease might be inside our brains, but the diagnosis will not change one life: it will change all of those around us.

The process of being diagnosed can be a lonely one. I attended each appointment on my own, even when the word 'dementia' had been lurking on too much paperwork to avoid any longer. But something cut through the shock of my final diagnosis to give me the foresight to ask the consultant if she would speak with my daughters directly. I left my girls to file into her office alone, looking as small as if they were still infants, knowing they would have questions for her that I couldn't answer, or ones that they were perhaps too mindful to ask in front of me. At that moment – just like anyone who is newly diagnosed – we didn't even know the right questions to ask, yet here was someone who potentially had the answers to the mystery that awaited us. It was at least a start, a chance to give my daughters the time and space to ask the things they needed to know. I was aware that this was their diagnosis as much as mine, that this disease would change their lives too.

The diagnosis process currently is far too clinical. The people who look inside our brains, and find connections are loose or missing altogether, dismiss us once they've found the root cause is a progressive disease. There is no follow-up, no coping strategies for me or anybody else. If I had been diagnosed with cancer, or a stroke, or diabetes, would the consultant have discharged me? So why is there no aftercare following diagnosis of a brain disease, and no continuing support?

There was no social support available – ironically, even less so for those with young-onset dementia. But there are so many husbands, wives, sons and daughters who are thrown into the new role of 'carer', the weight and expectation of society imposed immediately on them with no preparation, no planning, no warnings handed out alongside this life-changing diagnosis. No respect paid to the fact that these 670,000 carers within families for those with dementia save the NHS an estimated £11 billion every year. Given our increasingly ageing population, you would have thought they might be worth investing in.

I have been very vocal about the lack of aftercare for those of us with dementia and about what a difference it would make to our lives if we were prepared for all the eventualities that this disease may bring – many of them outlined in these very pages. But the same applies to our relatives, family and friends. If they too knew what might occur or if there was simply somebody to ask 'Is this normal?', they would be better prepared to deal with it. The solution is no more complicated than that, and it would lead to a better experience for both the person with dementia and those caring for them.

So when Dr Sahdia Parveen, researcher at Bradford University, asked if I would be on a project panel for her research, I was delighted to accept. The title of her project was the *Caregiving HOPE Study*, and it looked at the impact of a dementia diagnosis on the family of those who would be expected to care for that person. I am often asked to take part in research projects – it is a passion of mine because there is so much more that needs to be learned about this disease to give us a chance to outwit it – but Dr Parveen's work particularly appealed to me. She was interested in the juxtaposition between those who might feel culturally obliged to provide care for a relative or a parent, but were perhaps unwilling, and those who might be willing to care for a loved one, but might not be prepared for what that would involve in reality. It seemed to me that either of these two scenarios might be doomed to failure, so what could we do to understand them better?

Over the years I've come across many of these scenarios in real life, meeting couples where the wife resents her husband's dementia for ruining their old-age plans, to the daughter who so wants to look after her mum but is so exhausted from trying to navigate the scanty system of support that her own health has suffered. It's very rare to find people who have got the balance exactly right. But when you find these tiny pockets of inspiration, they are a joy to witness. One such woman I met had a husband with dementia and two young children, yet she was able to access daily support services that helped them all live a more balanced life. But the availability of this type of help, or of respite care, is so hit and miss.

According to statistics cited in Dr Parveen's report, in the future there will be a seven-fold increase in the number of people from South Asian communities (Pakistani, Bangladeshi and Indian) living with dementia, whereas the increase in the white British population is expected to be two-fold. A total of 723 carers completed the first questionnaire; of these 187 were South Asian and 522 were white British. While both demographics were equally willing to provide practical support, the report found white British carers were more willing to provide emotional support and nursing care. Tellingly, it was the white British carers who reported feeling more confident and also more prepared to care. The report found that 'feelings of cultural obligation to provide care were not associated with how willing carers were, or how prepared carers felt ... Better preparedness was associated with feeling more willing to provide care'. Preparedness was also 'found to be associated with more carer gains and lower burden, lower anxiety and lower depression'. So while white British people have less expectation on them, perhaps because they are able to *choose* to be carers, they feel more prepared for their role. Whereas cases where there is a higher level of expectation culturally does not make people feel more prepared for the role required of them.

Many of us do not discuss with our loved ones what our expectations are with regards to caring for one another until the moment is upon us. On the one hand, this is perfectly understandable – we're all busy getting on with life; I know I was – but as we can see from Dr Parveen's report, when people are more prepared they are also more willing and, crucially, more able to care.

ON HOW CARING CHANGES RELATIONSHIPS

Much of how you care will depend on the type of dementia someone has, but most importantly, a lot comes down to the type of person you are caring for. In ordinary life, we do change as we age – some of us can mellow, some can become more cantankerous – and it's certainly true that dementia adds another dimension to that melting pot of character. But the disease is still is only one facet of the person. You must see the person first and not the condition, just as you would for anyone else.

The difference between being prepared or not can be life-changing, both for the person with dementia and those caring for them. Look at these quotes from carers interviewed for Dr Parveen's report:

'It's really hard to know what a journey it's going to be, it's a good job that you don't know … You don't know how much you're going to get angry. I suppose anger – anger and guilt are the two things that I was least prepared for, and yet I knew, I knew in the abstract anger and guilt are around hugely, but to actually experience the anger and guilt, sometimes the anger towards her after repeat question after repeat question and I would say, "Oh shut up, you know I've told you a hundred times," and she doesn't understand, she can't help what she's saying. But I would say, "Oh shut up." That takes you by surprise. I still feel guilty about so many things; I could have done things so differently, I could have managed things so differently. I could have coped for longer with her aggression than I was doing, if I'd known then; if I'd known what was coming, I would never have had her admitted to hospital, I would never have agreed. I could have protected her in so many ways; there's so many shoulds around; I should have done something and yet here, in the end, you are only human.'

'People need to be prepared, they need to have an inner reserve of patience, and somehow recharge the batteries. I know it's difficult when you don't want to let go of somebody for a long period, but you need to … I used to have a couple of hours when one of her friends would come and take my wife out, and maybe I didn't recharge my battery in the right way at those times, maybe I rushed around and got some jobs done that it would've taken me days to to do with my wife, as they say, "in tow".'

There is a lot to be said for that old adage that tells us to apply our own oxygen mask before helping others. You are no use as a carer to anybody if your own energy supplies are run-down. Many carers spoke in Dr Parveen's report about how their own self-care strategies, such as having a coffee with a friend or getting their hair cut, helped them cope better in their roles as carers. That in turn benefits the person you're caring for.

Dementia changes relationships between couples for ever. Sometimes it is for the better: one woman I met in the course of my travels told me how her husband had often been violent in their marriage, and yet dementia had mellowed him and delivered her the husband she had hoped for all those years. For some it is, sadly, the opposite, and dementia can make behaviour more unpredictable and aggressive, particularly if you are living with a type of dementia such as Pick's disease.

I spoke to some of my friends about how their relationships have changed since diagnosis:

Wife: 'My relationship with my husband is better now than it's ever been; we're happier now. If I want something out of the oven because it's safer for him to do it, he comes straight away, whereas before it would be, "Oh, I'm busy." Now he helps me. I used to think I was a burden to my husband, but now I ask him because I know he doesn't mind.'

Husband: 'What annoys me is she will try and do things that she can't do. Instead of asking me straight away, she'll try and do it and get her knickers in a twist and then I'll have to sort it out. I wish she'd just let me do it. I wish she'd ask me straight away.'

Husband: 'My relationship with my wife has changed enormously. I tend to walk behind her now. I worry about saying and doing the wrong thing, but I'm very fortunate, as she's very good and makes sure I'm in the right place. I can still physically do the things I want to do – play tennis, walking and things. It's just those times when I think, where am I? What am I doing? and she'll bring me round.'

Wife: 'I wonder if that's a good thing, when you live with someone that you do things for them when they think they can't? I try to "support" rather than "do". We're still happy, we laugh, we have fun.'

Husband: 'We spend much more time with one another, which is generally good, but one of the difficulties for my wife is she can no longer go out of the house alone, even though we've lived here for forty years, because she gets disorientated. So if she wants to go somewhere, we always have to go together and that's a bit of a handicap.'

When people ask me how best to navigate relationships after a dementia diagnosis, I have only one answer: keep talking. I'll admit that it sounds simple in theory, and might not be so in practice, but that very much comes down to the individual.

I can still smell the air of my own kitchen, heavy with the scent of baking and sweet cakes that I had decorated in all different shapes and sizes, ready to sit down for that chat with my own daughters and discuss my power of attorney. That was my way of making that conversation just that little more palatable, but others will know what will work best in their own family.

Naively, I thought then that this awkward conversation would be a one-off. Perhaps I assumed we'd got the hardest conversation out of the way first as we sat down with pens and papers and cups of steaming tea, discussing everything from how I wanted to be cared for when I had tipped over the edge, to whether or not I would want to be resuscitated.

It was clear even then how differently my two daughters approached the same subject. I describe it as a talking exercise, but really it was a listening one. What I hadn't considered then was that this conversation would need to be repeated again and again as we were faced with new challenges.

We know from everyday conversations how confusing language can be. Even when you are speaking directly to someone, how many of our conversations result in crossed wires? When two people think they've been talking about the same thing in the same way, confusion can still reign. Add into the mix navigating a new future with a disease that is progressive and unpredictable, with its own rate of decline, and there are so many hazards to negotiate.

We are all guilty of making assumptions, even – and perhaps especially – with loved ones with whom we tend to speak in a kind of shorthand. That's why, when having conversations that are important to you, you need to be sure exactly what you are talking about. Something as simple as the term 'caring for a loved one with dementia' will mean one thing to one person and another to someone else. Caring is open to so many interpretations, and the word itself may need to be renegotiated over and over as time – and the disease – makes its march. For me, my need for 'care' means a time in my life when I'm no longer able to care for myself, when I physically and mentally can't find a way to keep living alone safely. My daughters both know that I don't want them to be my carers. I asserted that from the day I was diagnosed and I haven't changed my mind. I want my daughters to come and see me, to have a cup of tea, take me out for the day so that we can enjoy something together. But I don't want them coming to mine after a hard day's work and then having to sort my washing, or do my cleaning, or worse still, wash me. I want them to have their lives, and I don't want that life to be intruded on in any way that labels them as carers. I want to always be their mum, in whatever way that is possible. It's important to me to still feel useful to them, to care for them, even in a reduced capacity.

Dementia accelerates the process of role reversal. I do my best to avoid it. Before dementia my girls still came to me for advice, whether it was about something to bake or something to decorate. It happens less and less these days, but that doesn't mean I don't still cling on to the tiniest hint of my role as their mother. That is my primary job before anything else, including dementia, and I will guard it with everything I've got. I hate having to interrupt my daughters' busy lives to ask them for anything. I don't drive now, but wouldn't consider asking them for a lift anywhere unless I really can't get the bus or train. But if I'm honest, I do feel that the transaction is more one-sided than I would prefer these days. I remember one day not so long ago, when I was pegging out bed linen on my washing line and I suddenly thought of my daughter Sarah in her flat. She was working many extra shifts as a nurse and I realised it couldn't be easy to dry linen inside, so I worked out that there was something I could still do to help her. It felt so good to be able to ask her if I could do her washing each week. She did my heavy supermarket shopping for me, and somehow this evened things out. A mutually beneficial deal that was an ordinary thing for a mum to do.

For some cultures, as outlined in Dr Parveen's report, it's natural for ageing parents to be cared for by their adult children. Many generations of a family still live under one roof. But that often isn't the case in the West: many of us live apart and communities don't exist like they once did, so it can feel difficult to accept help from your children when you already know they have busy lives of their own. Even when they want to help out, it is difficult to agree to it. One of my friends living with dementia went so far as to persuade her daughter to move miles from her so that she wouldn't feel the need to become her carer. Her daughter already had a husband with a disability and two small children, so my friend didn't want to add to her burden.

For someone else, the term caring might mean helping out more generally. If you had a hundred people in a room, each would have a view of what caring meant. It could be doing intimate chores like washing someone and helping them in and out the bath, or it could be inviting them round for dinner – an expectation to include them in your day-to-day routine. Receiving care from a family member might not be appropriate, due to history within the family: they might not be close or there might exist long-held grudges. Likewise, those caring for family might be imposing their will on them without asking if the person with dementia wants to receive the care. I remember an anecdote from Dr Parveen's research where one lady of South Asian heritage received Tupperware boxes filled with curry from her family each night, but all she wanted to eat was fish and chips.

Caring is as individual as any family, and the term may have to be redefined many times over, as expectations or needs develop. Here are what people interviewed for Dr Parveen's report had to say:

'I do not want to be labelled as my mum's carer; I want to be my mum's daughter or, as my sister says, I want to just come and visit my mum and just go away. I want to just be the daughter I was, where I can just go and visit my mum, take her out for the day, have lunch, visit a nice house, not have to turn up, start doing washing, cooking, cleaning, making sure she's got social activities sorted out. I don't want to be labelled an official carer, but I feel, what choice do I have?'

'I just feel as if it's been forced upon me; half of me wants to be the good, chilled-out daughter that says, "But she's my mum and I will do it for my mum." These people who have had their parents live with them, I hold my hands up and say "all respect".'

ON CARING AS A DAUGHTER

There is no right or wrong reaction to being put into this position. It is as individual as the disease itself. My daughters and I have just had to feel our way through since my diagnosis. My daughter Sarah is an oncology nurse, but even for her, with her wealth of experience, it has not always been easy. I asked her to write a little for me on her own journey:

'Caring – that word has so many connotations,' Sarah writes.

I care, of course I care about Mum. Do I care *for* her? I'm not sure. Mum has said she never wants me to do any personal care for her – obviously I could do this, as it's a part of my job – however, this is one of Mum's main

wishes, and I can understand that. Instead it's a negoti-
ation; I make her meals, take her shopping, do some of
her cleaning, help her manage her finances at times and
organise and attend most health appointments. We go to
the coast and other beauty spots to take photos, which
is something she loves doing, and I visit or FaceTime
each day that I'm not at work. I don't consider most
of those tasks as any that are caring with a capital 'C'.
Quite the opposite, in some cases – many carers might
ask when would they get a chance to do any of the fun
things that we do – and anyway, most of them are things
I do frequently with other friends and family. For me,
that's just being a mum and daughter.

The difference, I guess, is that I probably don't worry
about other friends and family in quite the same way as
I do Mum. The potential for what might happen is the
bit that's changed – that low-level anxiety that you live
with each day. But I've had to learn not to let worry
and fear overwhelm me. When I'm nursing patients
at work, I'm all for positive risk-taking to improve
quality of life. However, within that there are constant
risk assessments, time constraints, and policies and
procedures which need to be in place to keep patients
safe in the ward environment. As a daughter of a fiercely
independent woman who will not be told what to do,
my work approach would not be suitable, so I have to
take off my work hat and leave it far behind, because
if Mum gets a hint that I'm reaching to put it on, I'm
outta there.

If anything, I've had to stop worrying about her.
We went to Italy for four days to speak at a dementia

conference and, during our time there, we got to spend some time sightseeing. One morning, we went with a guide for a short walk along a rocky path to a stunning viewpoint. Mum's gait has been affected by her dementia and she's now at a higher risk of falling, and at one point Mum tripped slightly but righted herself and carried on. Our guide commented on how relaxed I looked and how I wasn't rushing to grab Mum at any sudden movement. But I know my job as her daughter is to enable her to remain independent, and to do this, I have to let go of fear of what could happen. I used to constantly worry what would happen if she breaks a bone, hits her head, or worse. But, at the end of the day, if I had been stood by her side, wrapping her in cotton wool, she would not have had any joy in that walk. So now, I just think, whatever is going to happen, will happen. As long as there is joy, it's worth doing. I must admit, though, that sometimes I do walk in front of her so I can't see all her little stumbles.

I hear some sons and daughters talk of their experience and it seems as though the roles have been completely reversed, that they have become the parent. I don't feel that way. I've certainly had to become more responsible and available for Mum, but that's to help her live independently, not dependently. For anyone who is at the beginning of this journey, I would suggest stepping back and not jumping in to help. It took a lot of soul-searching for me to do that – it did not come naturally. When you love someone and you know you can do something for them, you just want to jump in and do it. But actually the most loving thing you can do is help them keep their sense of self by letting them be.

I'm reminded, when I read that from Sarah, of parenting her as a child, of those huge mountains we watch our children climb – heart in our throat, hoping they won't have an accident or fall. Yes, for some the roles have been reversed, but this is what they should be reversed to, that compassionate detachment that aids people's lives, not disables them.

How many times do we say to our young children, 'Be careful', 'Take care', 'Watch out', 'Do you think you should be doing that?' As parents we are continually on watch for accidents and mishaps, protecting those valuable little humans and wanting to shelter them from harm. But there comes a time for many of us when we realise we must let them make their own mistakes so that they can learn from them – or maybe not – and adapt their actions so the hurt is less likely. We need to give them space to have new experiences and adventures, and the freedom to try out new things with our full support. That's a safety net that most parents provide, giving children the freedom to learn from their own mistakes with the security of their parents' eyes on them if something goes wrong. Is it that different from caring for someone with dementia? as Sarah points out.

As a small child, Sarah lacked the confidence of others, but she was always desperate to try the things her friends were trying. I remember watching three-year-old Sarah at playgroup, all the mums sitting round in a circle, cups of tea in hand and the children playing in the middle of us all. There was a brightly coloured plastic climbing frame that had attracted her attention one particular day and she watched the others clamber and climb all over it, sliding down on the other side. Some mums were holding their children's hands as they gingerly stumbled and attempted what must have felt like a mountainous feat, but other mums blindly carried on chatting, only going to the rescue when things went wrong. Looking back, I think this was the first time as a parent that I realised that I had to let go of the fear of what *might* happen. How similar that is to what Sarah describes above.

I sat, half my attention on the chattering around me and half an eye on Sarah. I wanted to look away and let her work it out herself, but it was hard, just as it's hard for Sarah as an adult to let go of her fears about me. I didn't want her to see me watching and feel inhibited, so I glanced at her while pretending to watch the others as she figured out the safest route. I can still picture the concentration on her tiny face as, one rung at a time, gripping the sides, she pulled herself up, before finally reaching the summit. She stood there so proud, jumping up and down like the others and making a big noise, and it was only then that I allowed myself to be seen by her, my beaming smile matching hers.

I could have gone, like some parents did, and lifted their little ones straight up onto the platform – but where would the fun be in that? Would Sarah have felt that same sense of achievement? Sometimes, as parents, we just have to let our children take charge of their own experiences and make their own risk assessments. It's not always easy for parents, but now I see that it's not always easy for the adult children of those with dementia to let their parent do the same. In Sarah's case, by stepping back and not jumping in to help me, she allows me to live a more independent life and for that I am grateful. As Sarah said herself, where would the joy in life be if you were constantly being watched and told not to do something, or had others taking over and doing everything for you? It's so difficult for people to imagine – especially people who love us, like my daughters do. But by doing that, it gives us our life back. For me there is no greater gift than that.

ON LIVING ALONE

It is estimated that 50 million people live with dementia worldwide, and that is likely to increase to 152 million by 2050. In Canada, France, Germany, the UK and Sweden, more than a third to half of those living with dementia live alone, and generally, older women are the fastest-rising demographic of single-household populations in the world. Which means people like me. It makes sense to me that women of my generation, no longer restricted by the stigma of divorce, are choosing to live alone. But what does that mean when combined with an increasing number of us living with dementia?

Before dementia, there were times in my life when I wished that I hadn't felt so alone. I split with my husband in 1988, when my daughters were four and seven. After that, I raised them on my own. There were times in the intervening years before my dementia diagnosis when I wished there had been somebody else after him. There were days when work had been particularly tough and I just wanted someone with whom I could talk through a problem; someone who would put a supportive arm around my shoulders and tell me that everything would be all right. Or when a problem arose with one of the girls, it would have been nice to have been able to turn to someone and say: 'What do you think?' Or at weekends when I went out to eat alone and looked across at tables filled with couples deep in conversation. Or at night just to reach out and feel another body next to mine, to hear someone else's breath in the darkness.

Since my dementia diagnosis I have had those moments too: a back-up brain to jog my memory when I have forgotten an important date or an appointment somewhere would have been nice. Times when all you need is another human being sitting next to you to not feel lonely; that shortcut in language, a smile, a knowing look when words are unnecessary – those nuances of companionship that mean so much. A sense of safety to have someone at your side on days when life is a little frayed around the edges and has lost its sharp focus when you need to get from A to B. Someone with whom you can share something special that has occurred, like those times on my walks when I wish I could say: 'Did you just see that?' when a sparrowhawk swoops down and lands just feet in front of me. Someone to laugh with – *really* laugh. Sometimes, when I see other couples sharing a joke, I feel just like a teenager would, being left out of the crowd. I don't have someone to switch the cooker off when I forget, or someone who could have opened that Tupperware lid that defeated me the other day, which meant that instead of soup I made do with a sandwich for my tea.

Despite all this, it might surprise people to know that I feel I am better living with dementia alone.

I don't have someone rushing me or questioning. The one thing I always need more of is time. My brain can't work quickly, so the worst thing anyone can say to me is: 'Hurry up.' Those two tiny words prompt panic, confusion and a sense of failure. But living alone, my time is my own; I can go at my own speed.

I don't have someone questioning why I can't remember. That constant reminder of not remembering signals to me nothing but failure. 'Do you remember?' ... 'You *must* remember.' The constant twist of that knife. Now I don't answer someone when they say that to me, I just let them carry on. It's easier that way, otherwise they'll try and jog my memory with another detail that is just as insignificant to me. I often see couples, one partner adopting that tone of voice that says, 'I told you that yesterday,' the other looking lost and crestfallen at having to be told again, scolded like a child.

I don't have to give excuses for my actions. I can get things wrong and there's no big drama. I can come downstairs in the morning and find the bowl of food that I warmed the night before still in the microwave. I simply scrape it into the bin and wash the bowl. If someone else were there, they might be concerned that I'd missed a meal, or the waste, or the mess. For me it's just one of those things; better luck next time to remember that it is still in the microwave.

I don't have someone doing things for me because it's easier or quicker. No matter how long something takes me, it's always better to keep trying to do it myself. Dementia strips away so many tiny moments of independence that keep us feeling human, the last thing we want is to lose them all. I see it in couples all the time: the partners who are getting ready to leave and feel frustrated by how long it's taking their other half to zip their coat. 'Let me, it'll be quicker,' they say. Those five words are so disempowering. At least we have had our brains taken over by a disease; the other party is just allowing themselves to be influenced by impatience. If I get in a pickle trying to zip my coat one day, it's no big deal, I just go out without it fastened – I'll soon realise to snuggle it around me when I get cold.

I don't have someone fussing when I have a bad day. On those foggy days it's bad enough to have dementia in tow, let alone having someone else asking what's wrong or how to make it better – even if it is often for the kindest of reasons. If plans have to be changed, I never have to feel guilty for letting someone down. I remember one couple in particular: the wife telling me how they were due to visit friends for a coffee – people who they hadn't seen for ages, and she was so looking forward to it – but when the fog struck, her husband just wanted to stay at home, some-where without noise where he wouldn't have to chat and could sit in peace. His wife's disappointment was obvious, even as she recounted the story to me, and her husband's guilt was palpable. 'She should have gone without me,' he said. But she wanted to go as a couple.

I enjoy the fact that I don't have to talk if I don't want to. Silence is my friend, and my daughters know I love it. I am happy to be in their company and just not talk. At home, I can be silent for hours; no need to engage in conversation for the sake of it. I feel sorry for partners of those not wishing to speak. Having two humans in a house, it's natural to talk, but how lonely it must be to have someone next to you who feels unable to utter the words because it's so difficult to find the right ones. I would feel so incredibly guilty for denying someone a conversation.

I don't have to think whether I've upset someone. To think can often be exhausting, and to work out the possibility of having upset someone and why is no different. If I'm with my daughters, I know by their faces or tone of voice if I have upset them. I feel immediately sad and try to put it right in that moment. For couples, that thought from one day to the next of a long-forgotten (at least by one person) argument or unkind word might still linger in one of their hearts. That must be hard to reconcile. Or the resentment that can often be present between couples if one feels they are not understood, or their needs are not being met. It bleeds into every area of the relationship, and yet one person is oblivious. How do you say sorry when you've forgotten the reason you hurt someone? How does the partner without dementia forgive, when they may have already done that a thousand times?

I don't have to worry that I'm doing things differently. What does it matter if I have a cordless vacuum cleaner so I don't get tangled in the lead? It might not be as powerful, might not do as good a job, but it means I can still clean my house. If I were in a couple, my partner might insist on a proper vacuum cleaner, meaning I could no longer use it and then I would feel totally redundant – although, if I didn't enjoy hoovering, that might just work in my favour!

I don't have anyone correcting me when I say the wrong word, date, or name. I'm forever hearing partners correcting their loved ones when a name is wrong.

In the grand scheme of things, does it really matter? If you eavesdrop on a group of people with dementia, you will rarely hear corrections. Instead you will witness acceptance: people going with the flow. Putting someone right just leads to faltering, to hesitation while you double-check yourself, and then of course the flow of thoughts is lost.

I don't feel like I'm letting anyone down. That is my greatest gratitude in being single. We all make plans when we marry: to grow old disgracefully together, to have dreams of retirement, long country walks, wonderful holidays and other adventures. It's not until something happens to one partner that those dreams lie in tatters. I couldn't cope with that, with seeing the face of the person who was caring for me, their future stolen away alongside mine. It's often said that carers suffer and people with dementia live – I suppose we are in the here and now, whereas the partner can think of what might have been. When the disease progresses to the point when we would be unrecognisable to the person we are now, we won't even be aware of the heartache, trauma and suffering caused.

Living alone, I *have* to find a way around the challenges of my day-to-day life. Is this what keeps my dementia at bay, the very fact that I am single? I couldn't live alone if I hadn't faced all my challenges and found ways around them. It's that determination to stay living alone, to keep finding solutions, that helps me outwit dementia every day.

I have a real problem with people coming into my house now. I find it difficult, as I'm not used to it; it seems strange and alien to me, so I wouldn't be a prime candidate for accepting home care – it would leave me feeling disorientated to have someone popping in. Many people living on their own have developed their own routines and would find it disconcerting to have to adapt to the ways of a live-in carer. I asked two of my friends recently how they would feel about live-in help. 'Anxious' was the word they used: they couldn't imagine someone being understanding enough to accept them as they were, who would be willing to understand *their* dementia, and not expect them to accept *their* way of caring.

ON THE NEED FOR CONNECTIONS

There are benefits to living alone. But that's not to say that you don't sometimes feel the pinch of loneliness at the lack of relationships around you.

A 2019 Cambridge University Press report looked into how those living alone sought relationships – even if that was only brief encounters – in their community. These meetings, whether planned or spontaneous, provided meaningful contact, which reportedly made participants of the study feel safer and less alone in their neighbourhood. I know how they feel: on days when I feel particularly isolated, I often time my own walks in the hope of bumping into other villagers. It's amazing what a simple hello or a smile can provide if you see no one else in your day, and this doesn't just apply to people with dementia, but to all of us – I know many villagers who do the same. I adore living alone, but I do find myself increasingly lonely and need that human contact to prove to myself that I can still talk; that people will still engage with me; that I exist. I don't get the companionship from the TV that some speak of – a human smile is far more fulfilling to me than an electrical appliance in the corner of the room – so I go for a walk to seek out that human connection.

People interviewed as part of the study mentioned how even a brief chat on the staircase of their communal flats made them feel more connected, and that 'neighbours provided a low but consistent level of daily support'. This support is important because it can fend off feelings of isolation that lead to depression. People reported how they felt safer because they sensed that these people who they had regular contact with also kept an eye on them. However tenuous their link to them – they might just be the owner of a local café they visit – they still felt that if they didn't turn up for a few days, that person might raise the alarm.

The truth is unavoidable: people who live alone with dementia are more prone to unplanned hospitalisations and malnutrition; they are admitted to long-term care at an earlier point to others; they are less well connected to formal services and lack the advocacy of a co-resident carer. So we do need support to help us live alone, and if that support does not come from within our families, it comes from friends and neighbours or the wider community. But, as many of my friends point out, friendships change after dementia. In the 2019 report, a 79-year-old Swedish woman spoke of how her existing social circle shrunk, which in turn made her feel isolated. The problem, she explained, was the lack of understanding about dementia within her friendship group, which meant that they didn't understand that she couldn't remember their regular meeting places any more. This lead to her feeling shamed by her disease and withdrawing from that group.

It was definitely like that for me in the beginning, and it's still the same now when I meet people for the first time and they know I have dementia. I have to confront the fears that I see on their faces, and disrupt them with my personality and conversation. Sometimes it takes longer – their disbelief being a barrier to their acceptance of me as I am – but I can usually persuade people to see me as a person first and then see the dementia. It's when they see my dementia first that it can take some time.

Another friend of mine had a similar experience after she was diagnosed. She told me how her friends have slipped away and that makes her sad because they've been good friends for many years, but they don't understand that the woman on the outside isn't the same woman they knew on the inside. She feels lost and left out. Her husband explained this to me:

'My wife's friendships have just fallen away since her diagnosis. Six of her friends have been widowed in this last year, so they've formed a group amongst themselves, but she can't process conversations quickly so she's excluded from the group. She finds it very sad as they've been friends for years.'

Another friend who has dementia put it like this:

'I was always the organiser, the chair of the WI, delivered art classes, etc. I don't feel that I belong now, I'm not a part of things any more. It hurts. I was much more confident before and am not as capable of being as organised since dementia.'

Her husband agreed: 'It's not the partner and children who are the issues, it's friends and making new friends. Having the confidence to get into new friendships and groups has gone. Sue's found it very difficult to find that confidence. Lack of friends is the biggest issue.'

The 2019 report recognised that, sadly, social losses seem to be a part of a lot of people's lives post-diagnosis. The authors put this down to three things: a lack of social awareness of what dementia means; a lack of acceptance of the condition; and a lack of compassion for those living with the disease. The report concluded that support services within communities are key to building awareness and making neighbourhoods more dementia-friendly, as well as providing much-needed contact to avoid those living with dementia feeling isolated and therefore prone to depression. But in England and Scotland, with public-sector services in decline, it is often left to voluntary organisations to fill that void. Ten years ago, there apparently used to be a Young Dementia service in the East Riding where I live, but it was disbanded a year or two before I was diagnosed because the need wasn't there. It's important that we don't only rely on voluntary organisations to do the work that the public sector should be doing. Some support needs specially trained people, and charities can't always afford to employ them. Support immediately post-diagnosis is the most important way to try and enable people to build resilience and to remind them that there is still a life to be lived. In Scotland, everyone newly diagnosed receives a support worker for a year who can direct them to services, but after that year the support is withdrawn.

The Cambridge University Press report recommends that there be 'more opportunities for social meeting places in neighbourhoods which help to overcome generational divisions and increase knowledge about dementia'. It says: 'A litmus test for emerging dementia-friendly community initiatives will be the extent to which those who live alone with the condition are enabled to thrive and participate in their local communities alongside their peers and neighbours.'

I agree with that. If we're embraced by a community as a human being, just like everyone else, we will thrive and feel part of something bigger – and I do believe communities will feel better as a result of it. Everyone has their challenges; mine just happens to be dementia.

ON PEOPLE WITH DEMENTIA AS CARERS

The number of women living alone with dementia may be rising, but there is another demographic of people who are becoming more common, and that is the number of people living with dementia themselves who are also caring for someone with the disease. With a rising population of people being diagnosed, it is inevitable that this will be the reality for some. A good friend of mine, Agnes Houston, is one of them.

I met Agnes when I heard her speak at a conference in 2015 – almost a year after my own diagnosis with dementia. I was impressed with her positive attitude and how she was determined that there was still so much living to be done with this disease in tow. From that moment onwards, we have become firm friends, both of us regular speakers, activists and advisers on many committees. In her life pre-dementia, Agnes was an intensive-care nurse, which you would think would prepare her for the situation she finds herself in. But caring for people professionally and within your own family are two very different things.

Agnes was diagnosed with dementia in 2006. Her husband, Alan, was diagnosed a few years later, but looking back, Agnes wonders whether his own disease lay undiagnosed for years before that. He certainly couldn't cope when she was diagnosed with dementia, and after becoming increasingly irresponsible with their money, which on reflection was a manifestation of his symptoms, the couple decided to live separately. Agnes is helped at home by her own support worker, but she is still fighting for a care package for Alan, and in the meantime she is his main carer.

'If I hadn't been a nurse, I would be dead and Alan would be in care,' Agnes explains. 'You can get some kind of satisfaction for caring for someone who is physically dependent, but with caring for someone with dementia, you've got to dig really deep to get satisfaction.

'Alan doesn't realise he's in danger. He acknowledges his dementia verbally – he's very proud of the fact he has two dementias: vascular and Alzheimer's – but he doesn't understand the disease on a deeper level. If he acknowledges its full extent, he sees his lack and he doesn't want to be reminded of what he can't do.

'I don't like the word "carer", but I know we need to use it. I have different roles: as a carer, a nurse, a wife.

You have to break it down into physical care, psychological care and cognitive prompting. For example, I don't need to physically put Alan in the shower, but he wouldn't have a shower if I didn't tell him, and he'd put the same clothes on if I didn't take the dirty ones. I have to monitor his hydration, his intake of food, especially because he lives alone; even though he has microwave meals, he finds it easier to make a sandwich, but he'll eat a whole loaf and that's not good for you. Also, he tells me what I want to hear – he'll tell me he had this beautiful meal, and I'll say, "Well, where did you get the chicken from? I didn't bring a chicken to you," but then he'll try and convince me I did buy chicken and it's my dementia – until I go and check in the bin. It's very tiring for me.

'In any marriage, one partner can end up compensating for another, but with dementia, if you start over-compensating for them, then you're disempowering them. For example, Alan doesn't understand the value of money any more, so I have to give him the exact money so he can go and get his newspaper. It just becomes so complicated that you think, "I won't bother – I'll just order his paper to be delivered," because it's just too difficult, but then you're disempowering them by doing it for them. My support workers even try to do the same for me, and you have to be a really strong character not to let someone do things for you. But if you let people put your gloves on, or put your hat on, before you know it, you can't dress yourself. But I've done it myself: if you need to get someone to a doctor's appointment on time, you might end up buttoning their jacket, and so disempowering them.

'I pick my battles with Alan. I remember one day he was having his tea and he got up and I said: "What are you doing now, darling?" because I'm frightened he will fall, and he said: "I'm getting the ladder out; if the ladder is there I will remember I have something to do with the ladder." And so it sat there, and it was doing my head in. I couldn't remember why it was there, and eventually I said: "Darling, we've finished with the ladder, would you put it away now?" We should be in a sitcom – nobody would believe it.

'I just thought what I was doing for Alan was what a wife would do, but as a carer and a person living with dementia, I have to realise that I have needs as well and they're being neglected. I want to get a package of care to meet Alan's outcomes and that will lift the rucksack off my back, so I don't have to do all this medical management and I can just be his wife. Agencies have not got the capacity to take in that I have dementia as well. I am doing their job for them.'

I asked Agnes if, aside from the desperate need for more care for Alan, there was anything that would help couples who are both living with dementia.

'We need couples therapy,' she said. 'Alan's got his struggles with dementia, and I've got my struggles with dementia, and I can only see it through the prisms of my glasses and Alan can only see it through the prisms of his glasses and how he's looking at the world. It would be nice to get an insight, not to play a blame game, but to understand each other better; for example, he could say, "If you left the ladder there it would help me," instead of us fighting over the ladder. I can't see the issues we have, and

Alan hasn't the ability to tell me what they are. But given time and different ways of trying to get the information out of him, then we might have that light-bulb moment and then we could put solutions in place, and I wouldn't have to disempower him, which would relieve a lot of stress.'

I can't imagine how hard it is for Agnes to keep having to remind herself to put her own needs first, when her instinct is to care for others. I know of another couple in sheltered accommodation, both of them living with dementia, and when the husband went into hospital recently, doctors were so keen to discharge him from their care that they didn't understand why his wife was unable to make arrangements for him to come home. Another friend of mine all the way over in New Zealand has dementia, and she has been a carer for her physically disabled husband for the last twenty-five years. Yet she told me that now, for the first time in more than two decades, their relationship has evened itself out, with each of them providing care in different ways for the other.

Just as with any relationship, it takes constant nego-tiation and give and take. Dementia just adds another element to the equation.

COMMUNICATION

How vital are words to our need to communicate? I can still see each of my daughters as babies, sitting up in high chairs, feeling very proud of themselves as they took their first bites of a banana. They babbled along as they did, the sounds and gurgles indecipherable, yet – like all mothers – I answered them as if what they said made perfect sense to me. When they were a bit older and learned the word 'yes', we could go backwards and forwards in conversation for hours, as long as I asked the right questions. But it wasn't always a verbal answer that they needed from me. A mother and child communicate in all sorts of ways, nurturing with smiles and nods, a squeeze, or a laugh to match their own. My girls will testify that as they grew older, they also grew more adept at this non-verbal communication of ours. There were the good times when all they needed was a reassuring nod from me from across the school field on sports day to give the next race all they'd got, or a smile when they were perched on a high wall that they were trying to build the courage to leap from. There were also the times when a raise of my eyebrows was enough to warn them that whatever they were about to attempt next would be met with disapproval, or when my appearance at their bedroom door, just a sideways glance, was all they needed to know that it was time to put whatever they were arguing about to bed.

It is said that only 7 per cent of our communication is verbal. Fifty-five per cent of it is body language and 38 per cent is tone of voice. I know that as I sat with my dying mother, there was no need for any words at all. The touch of my hand on hers in that moment said everything there was left to say. She just needed to know that I was close, and that she wouldn't be alone when death finally came to claim her.

In the animal world, words aren't necessary: there are purrs and licks, and a nose from a new mum is often enough to keep her new brood in line. Why do humans, then, place so much stock in words, when most of the time there are never enough of them to say what we really feel inside?

Before dementia, I enjoyed long dinners, sitting in restaurants, conversation bouncing back and forth between courses. But, as I have already explained, after my diagnosis the clanging of cutlery, the background noises and my inability to keep up with conversations meant that I retreated from the table. I sat back in my chair, just content to listen. Did my silence mean that I wasn't contributing? Perhaps. But did my chair around the table make me still feel included? Most definitely.

Communication comes in all shapes and forms. When dementia cruelly affects the power of speech or even steals it away completely, it's other people that can often make the wrong choice to stop talking to us or stop visiting – to stop giving us a chair at the table. They don't think of all that non-verbal expression, that essential currency we use to communicate with others throughout our lives – a glance between husband and wife that says a thousand words, the concern in their voice when it's been a tough day. Why would someone with dementia, who is no longer able to speak in the way they once did, not need that any more?

I remember participating in some research at York University, along with others living with dementia. One of them was Maria Helena, who has sadly passed away now. She was originally from Colombia and attended the study alongside her husband. She was further along in her dementia journey than many of us but enjoyed the conversation just as much as we did. How did I know? It is true that her verbal skills weren't what they used to be and that she kept lapsing into her native Spanish, but she connected with the researcher, hugging her and laughing along with the rest of us even when she couldn't find the words. That was *her* contribution to the research, and the day wouldn't have been the same without her.

I understand that it can be upsetting for people who visit their loved ones in care homes and find that they are no longer recognised. I know the pain that causes, and for me, that is my biggest fear: the moment when my girls are faced with the very same hurt and pain. I do not belittle it at all. But we need to remember that all of us go through life communicating with people in ways that don't involve speech; we can all think of a time in our lives when non-verbal communication was all we needed for care or reassurance. I find the thought that someone would give up on talking to me just because I could no longer talk back very sad indeed. Try telling an intensive-care nurse who spends hours beside an unconscious patient that they are suddenly devoid of personality, of likes and dislikes, of wants and needs.

One of my American friends has lost the ability to speak. She was a journalist in her former life, and it seems so cruel that dementia would snatch the ability to speak from her of all people. Yet the part of her brain that uses the keyboard is still very much alive inside her. She can still write, so eloquently and with so much emotion, yet she cannot say the words she longs for people to hear. Does that mean she should be excluded from joining in? Should her silence make others feel uncomfortable when it's clear that inside there is still so much that she wants to say? She is further down the path than me, but I find it comforting that she still possesses that skill to communicate. Outwardly she might seem lost, a vacant, speechless being, yet not only does she type, but she often paints how she feels as well. Her paintings are as evocative as the thoughts that must race round her head. Does it matter that she cannot speak when this is not the only way we go on our way through this world?

My friend Christopher Devas is now sadly in the later stages of his disease and has lost the ability to speak, yet he still loves to attend his choir. When he stands there and the music of a song he loves starts up, he will sing the words as if the power of his day-to-day voice had never left him. He stands proud, singing from his heart, the melody running through his veins, indelible. There have been other stories that have gone viral, like the emotional clip of former prima ballerina Marta Cinta González – who sadly died in 2019 – listening to a recording of Tchaikovsky's *Swan Lake*, which she danced to in her youth. There, in front of the camera, the music worked its way into her muscle memory and she started moving and swaying as elegantly as she had in her pre-dementia days. Or the story of Paul Harvey, an eighty-year-old man living with dementia who, in his former career, was a concert pianist and composer. His son recorded him composing the most beautiful piece of music using just four notes, which sped to the top of the iTunes charts.

'My memory's fine when I'm playing the piano,' he told the *Guardian*. 'I can remember all the things I've done. When I am looking at the television or other things around where I live, then I start forgetting things. And if something is not in the right place, then I panic a bit. But if I'm stressed, I will go and play the piano, and I'll be all right then.'

I have said countless times that we all had talents before our dementia diagnosis, and we don't suddenly lose them overnight. My friend Monica from the Minds and Voices group I attend in York always plays the piano for us at the end of our hour-long Zoom calls – a beautiful classical piece that leaves us feeling at peace. She used to be a music teacher long before dementia entered her world, yet even though dementia is a companion now, it isn't clever enough to steal those wonderful musical notes from her.

The way I speak now is not what it once was. Sometimes I cringe to hear a recording of myself: that hesitancy in my voice – even the sound of it; the pause while I search for simple words that escape me. When I give speeches I have to read them from a printed sheet of paper. I always start my monologue explaining that if I didn't have notes in front of me, I would lose the thread and my mind would veer off into all sorts of subjects not relevant to the topic.

Some have criticised me for that, saying that this act in itself does little to reflect my dementia, but time is so limited on those occasions that I always want to make sure all my points are made.

I can understand that for some this frustration at not being able to speak as we once did becomes too much, that those words and thoughts that escape us like butterflies, sometimes impossible to pin down, are simply exhausting, and that it's better just to give in and stay silent. We had a friend at Minds and Voices who came along to every session, yet chose to stay silent each week. One day we separated off and I sat with her in the corner of the room, sharing a cup of tea and not much more. There was no pressure in that time we spent together for either of us to talk. I hoped that would make her feel relaxed, to have somebody by her side simply for the pleasure of it instead of trying to coax shy words from her. I noticed through her body language how her confidence increased in smaller settings. She started to understand that my friendship came without expectation, and so when she finally tried to utter a string of words, I waited without hurrying her. There was no embarrassment when I didn't understand her, nor were there any uneasy moments. What did it matter if I didn't grasp each word? What was more important was the connection that we shared. Laughter was our substitute in that moment. How many times have you shared a moment of humour with somebody else that bound you closer than any words might do? It was the same with us. We both had dementia, we both understood, and that allowed her the freedom not to worry: to simply be.

If you spend enough time with someone, you can read them like the proverbial book. One friend, whose husband had dementia and has since sadly passed away, said she could tell how he felt or what sort of day he was having – good or bad – simply by the expression on his face. Loved ones know each line and crease of their relative's face so well that care-home or hospital staff should pay more attention to what they are able to intuit. My mind flashes forward sometimes, mostly in nightmares, but sometimes simply in curiosity, to a time when I might not be able to say what it is that I want. I hope the bonds of love that have bound me and my daughters so tightly, since the days they sat up in their high chairs and told me stories that I tried so hard to understand, will serve me well in those later stages. That when the time comes, and I can no longer speak the words, my daughters can read from my eyes what I want and need.

No one knows what people with dementia are really thinking in those later stages or how they really feel when they can no longer speak the words. Are they still capable of those thoughts, just as someone trapped in a malfunctioning body or deep in a coma can sometimes hear all that's being said around them? If that's what awaits me, I'd like to think that my two girls – those who I love the most – will be there to keep me company with the sound of a voice I know so well, or a touch of the hand, and they will know intuitively how happy that will make me, even if the words escape me.

ON FACING CRITICISM

My blog, *Which Me Am I Today?*, attracts visitors from all over the world. I have more than 4,000 regular visitors from places as far-flung as Australia, South Korea, Russia, Mexico and Myanmar.

It started off simply as my memory, a way of remembering what I did each day, and it still is. I was lucky that I foresaw the importance of keeping a record of my memories when living with a disease that would steal them from me as I slept. But as I learned more about my disease, I realised that there was another meaning to my blog: it was a place to share ideas and information. As people started following me and commenting, I saw the need and desperation for this very same information, and how grateful people were to receive it:

'Wendy, let me start by saying that I look forward to your posts on a daily basis. I think my mum has the beginning of dementia, but unlike you she won't go for a memory test. I want to understand what it is like to have dementia and some of the things you have said I have already been able to use with my mum. Please keep writing these blogs – they are both comforting and inspiration.'

'Thank you, Wendy. I feel stronger and more informed. My husband has just been diagnosed with cognitive impairment and I feel I know a little more about the disease now. It's very hard both for the patient and for the carer.'

'Wendy, my dad and both brothers all had dementia. However, my lovely husband and I have talked about what you have written and I feel less afraid now for the future should either of us be diagnosed. You don't make light of dementia, but give sound principles for survival and even moments of joy.'

'My husband has advanced Alzheimer's and reading about your journey is so helpful in understanding the progression of this disease.'

When spoken language started to fail me, I found that writing my blog was an escape from the roadblocks in my mind. For some reason, the frustration with words didn't exist between my mind and the page. Here, at my keyboard, I didn't stumble in my search for a phrase; somehow the process of my fingers dancing across the keys meant the words came more fluently. There was a time early on when I had not typed for a few days. I thought this respite would be a welcome break for my hands, but when I returned to the keyboard, my fingers no longer knew what to do with themselves. I stared at the blank screen and then tried typing – nothing I pressed made sense. Letters appeared, but not in any order. I was terrified that I had lost this ability of mine, the one that always cut through the fog, and from that day on I have never let a single day go by without typing again. Typing has become my escape from dementia; a part of my day when I look at the screen and see normality staring back at me. It's a daily freedom that overrides my ailing brain, as if my grey matter is taking scenic country lanes to avoid the traffic jams on major roads. The hesitant verbal me can feel frustrating, but the typing me feels calm, fluent and closer to my thoughts and feelings. If I didn't have that ability to type, I'd be lost, caught up in the hesitancy and inability to express myself.

I understand that it must come as a surprise to some people who read my blog to see me in person if I am not reading from a pre-prepared script. They are probably expecting someone far more eloquent to who I am in the flesh. There are also those who think that people like me – dementia activists, if you like – are giving a false impression of what this disease really represents. Some eminent names have gone so far on social media to cast their doubts on our diagnoses, and their abuse can be hurtful and devastating to our confidence. Anyone knows that once you put your head above the parapet to speak about a topic, you are opening yourself up to a certain amount of criticism. I remember one of the first events I attended, where a small group of people sat around a table discussing dementia and what it meant for them. Those days were the early ones of my own diagnosis, and I could perhaps speak with more eloquence than I can now. But as we went around the table and I had finished saying whatever it was that I wanted to say, another man piped up that his own mother had 'real dementia' and looked at me as if I were in some way faking it – forgetting, as people tend to do, that this disease has a beginning and a middle, as well as an end.

I have faced a lot of criticism like this over the years since my diagnosis. It still hurts me on weak days and I feel like I just want to hide away this 'typing me', to take it off and give the critics what they want. Soon, though, their comments fade into insignificance, overridden by my love of – and need for – typing.

People fail to take into account just what it takes out of me to push myself to try. At talks, people have often said, 'It's all right for you,' when they see how I can communicate sitting up there on the stage, but what they won't see is the banging headache that might hang around for days afterwards simply because of the exertion of attending that event, or all the planning that goes into arriving there in the first place. They seem to think I just appear, but in reality my planning starts weeks in advance: plotting my route, printing out images of landmarks I might pass on my way so that it will feel more familiar when I get there. People simply don't consider the energy it takes to arrive in front of them. They don't see me curled up in bed the next day, my head unable to even gauge even which day of the week it is, simply because I have exhausted myself. But what choice do I have? To stay at home and not speak out at all? Would that make people feel better? Would they prefer I left it to the 'experts' to talk about this disease that wreaks havoc in my brain, rather than hear it from me?

It is these very same 'experts' that question whether our initial diagnosis was correct if we do not follow the traditional trajectory of this disease. I remember one friend being so affected by the doubt and hurtful remarks that she never went on Twitter again. Another friend even went back to her consultant and asked for a second opinion, so bullied was she on social media, that she wondered if her own brain was playing tricks on her. Both NHS resources and her own emotional energy were wasted in this exercise, which of course only produced the same result. I haven't allowed myself to be bullied into that position. It was tragic enough the first time around – why should I go through it again just to satisfy someone else's curiosity and disbelief? But I know being able to type and write often works against me, as it gives people a warped perception of my life. Maybe, in its own way, this is a gift from dementia, and considering that this disease grants so few of them, I will not let it slip. Often I am just as astounded by the dance my fingers make across the keyboard and the sentences that they produce as anyone else. There is little – if any – research in this area to explain why this part of my brain still functions when so much is failing. No one is able to give me an explanation.

Perhaps if professionals concentrated more on what we can do from the start, our lives would be so much more hopeful from the point of diagnosis. Professionals often see people in the later stages and so find it difficult to understand people in the early stages. Many misjudge us because of this lack of knowledge, which can lead them to doubt our diagnosis. We often say: 'Live in our shoes for twenty-four hours and you may change your mind about questioning it.' Yet people can't do that. They will never see what our real lives are like, our day-to-day life with dementia, but while I'm still able to, I'll continue to write about it.

ON THE FACT THAT WORDS MATTER

When it comes to communication, we cannot be expected to take responsibility for the way others describe us – no matter how inaccurate it is. It starts, of course, right back at that first point of diagnosis with the language that is used. As I said at the start of this chapter, words are important, but so are images, metaphors – all the ways that we communicate with one another. When I was first told that I had dementia, the image that appeared in my mind was that of a white-haired old lady lying in a hospital bed. I looked in the mirror; that wasn't me. I couldn't relate to her. Where did this image come from? Who had put it there in the first place? We don't notice the slow, insidious effect of language and images that we come across every day through society or the media. This doesn't just affect the perception of the general public, but that of professionals too – perhaps that is why they present dementia at diagnosis as something terminal that can't be treated, rather focusing on it simply as a new way of living.

Dementia can be described as a journey, although there has been a question mark over how accurate that is when a progressive illness is not something that you can come back from. Journey is an odd word. I don't like to use it, but sometimes I can't think of anything else to use. Journeys, after all, are something I undertake with relish. 'My journey to paradise' is the way I describe my regular visits to the Lake District. Journeys are something I have chosen to take, with destinations that I look forward to arriving at, which is obviously not the case when I think of dementia.

Likewise, take describing dementia – or perhaps any serious illness – with the language of war: that it is a 'battle' to be 'fought' implies that if you don't win, you must surely be a loser. But how can that be the case when your 'enemy' is a progressive illness? You really would be fighting a losing battle. The public continually describe us as fighting and battling when all we simply want to do is to live the best we can. It can make people feel like a failure if they're not 'willing to go to war'. For example, the way that I go about my life and the effort I put into 'outwitting' my dementia is a daily challenge, one that I find exhausting and that other people may not want to take on. Does that make them a failure and me a fighter? No. We're just choosing to deal with this disease in different ways. It is also not at all helpful to think of dementia as a 'death sentence', which I know is something that a lot of people describe it as – perhaps even I did internally in those early days. Referring to dementia in these terms has nothing but negative connotations.

The fact of the matter is that each individual has the right to describe their own condition, exactly as they see fit, but what they hear from others is important. A 2016 paper, 'Ethical Implications of the Perception and Portrayal of Dementia', aimed to establish just how much language affected the perceptions of dementia, not just from the public's point of view, but also for those who were living with the disease. The report recognised that for some, particular language is useful – for example, the word 'journey' gave them hope or helped them cope – but for others it summed up a sense of dread or loss of self. Progress is being made all the time, as the report outlined.

> Over time, the use of words changes to avoid the nega-
> tive connotations that develop from association with a
> condition that is still negatively valued; for example,
> 'senility' being replaced by 'dementia'. Just as each
> term carries an ethical dimension, so each change can
> bring and foster a fresh perspective. For example, being
> labelled 'a dement' married the person with the term
> and removes personhood; 'being demented' implies
> that a person with dementia is only this; 'living with
> dementia' implies that one can still have a life with
> dementia.

My least favourite word is 'suffer', and unfortunately this is the one that is used most often to describe someone living with dementia – a sufferer. I always challenge this, particularly when I'm speaking to trainee nurses heading out into the world to work with people who are living with dementia. 'Do I look like I'm suffering?' I ask them, and they have to admit that I do not. If you were described that way, day after day, you might start to believe it.

Here's what some of my friends have to say about the use of language and how it affects them:

'You hear a lot about suffering, lots of what we're not capable of, but we're not stupid, we're just not able to reply as easily as we did; it takes us time and we can go blank about how to say things and what to reply, and it gets you frustrated and it can be frightening. The family has realised that one-to-one chats are much better than a group chat.'

'I can't keep up when people talk fast, and especially on the television and if there's a crowd of you in church and lots of people are talking, I can't hear what anyone is saying; they all jumble together. We're not stupid and we can do things. Healthcare professionals have got to get in their minds that you mustn't try and change people with dementia. They're the same person as before they were diagnosed.'

'Negative language makes me very withdrawn. As much as I try, when I do see my friends, because of my Alzheimer's, it's like having a monkey on my back. I don't know if it's because they find it difficult, but I started not to go out with friends because I didn't feel part of it and that made me sad. I would like to think it if had been one of them, I hope I would have had a talk and asked if there's anything we can do, but nobody said anything to me. It's very strange.'

ON LANGUAGE USED BY PROFESSIONALS

In 2019, Professor Dawn Brooker, a clinical psychologist, was invited to give a speech to the Faculty of Older People within the British Psychological Society. In it, she talked about her experience of how the way dementia is seen within the medical profession has changed over the course of her career. In the eighties, she said:

> … the language used by professionals was often hideous and reinforced negative stereotypes and connotations … Similarly, the nursing staff called the older people's in-patient ward the 'babies ward'. One of my greatest achievements was getting the name of the overarching service I was part of changed from 'Elderly Severely Mentally Infirm' to 'Mental Health Services for Older Adults'.

She went on to talk about how back then psychologists were aware that the carer of the person with dementia had needs, but 'the prevailing attitude was that people with dementia did not have emotional needs. Medical professionals thought they couldn't feel pain, and ingrained within every service was the feeling that dementia was the "empty shell that left the body behind".'

The cultural shift, she said, came with the work of Tom Kitwood, who enabled people to see the person behind the diagnostic label. His dementia-care model is still in use today. This model put love at the very centre of the work that a carer does, but also highlighted the importance of occupation (having a purpose in life), comfort (being free from distress and pain), identity (a sense of who we are), inclusion (a feeling of belonging), and attachment (a feeling of security and safety).

Professor Brooker agreed that Kitwood's model changed the way that she worked, and concluded her speech by saying: 'People with dementia have found their voice within society, but Kitwood's work has made professionals and researchers in this field more willing to hear and indeed amplify that voice.' She admits that there is still a long way to go but says: 'Our aspirations and expectations of what is acceptable and possible have changed for the better, but if we keep love at the centre of our work, we can only continue to improve.'

I hope it's now accepted that dementia is not a mental illness but a neurological condition, although many occurrences make me doubt that hope. It may affect a person's mental health, but the condition itself is a disease of the brain, not a faulty brain chemistry. We're placed under the remit of mental health services of older adults, regardless of our age – so you could be diagnosed with young-onset dementia at fifty and find yourself sitting alongside an eighty-year-old. I've heard of some people not wanting to go for a diagnosis because the disease is associated with mental health, and unfortunately there is still a huge stigma about mental health in society. But, as you can see from Professor Brooker's speech, progress is being made, even if it is in tiny incremental steps.

The psychological effect of words and body language must never be underestimated by anyone, particularly by professionals. How different my mindset would have been if I had left my neurologist's office after that initial diagnosis with a better choice of words ringing in my ears — sending me away with hope of a life instead of despair. The same is true of the PIP (Personal Independence Payment) process, which seems to penalise us for our attempts to stay as active as we possibly can, and focuses instead on what we cannot do to establish whether we are eligible to receive financial assistance from the government. That's why so many of us struggle to complete the forms: we are so busy concentrating on what we can do that we tend to forget what we can't do any more. Yet this process stresses the negatives without taking into account the strategies we've come up with to cope with tasks.

It is hard to get it right for everyone, and this is something the 2016 report acknowledges. 'Where there is fear of naming dementia due to its negative connotations, euphemisms may be coined which in themselves carry ethical dimensions. For example, the description of services as "memory clinics" may allow some to attend without a sense of stigma but may also deter those with different early symptoms from seeking help.'

The name 'memory clinics' has long been criticised because dementia isn't just about memory, so that implication in itself gives people the wrong idea. Some people with dementia actively call themselves a 'dementia sufferer', which is fine if that's what they want to call themselves. But choice is really what it's all about. It's the same reason why I don't like the phrase 'living well with dementia'.

Some years back it felt like a good idea because there was nothing else other than 'suffering', but I've since realised from meeting so many other people that the phrase itself sets a high standard that not everyone can reach, and so can end up having a negative effect. It leaves some people feeling inadequate, given that many days are simply rubbish days. How can anyone live well through those?

I remember meeting one chap at one of my talks whose whole demeanour was very sad. His head drooped and he exuded defeat. He came to talk to me afterwards, saying he wanted to wish me well. We chatted for a few minutes, about this and that, and he told me that he too had been diagnosed with dementia.

'How are you coping?' I asked him.

'It's rubbish,' he said. 'I could never do what you do, it's too late for me.'

This time the sadness reached his eyes.

'Why?' I asked. 'Why is it too late? You look to me as if you're at the same stage as me, unless I'm wrong?'

'I just hate that phrase "living well",' he told me. 'I'm forever hearing it's possible to live well, and then I just ask myself, why can't I?'

'Then we'll have to think of a new phrase,' I told him, 'because I don't want to be responsible for you feeling sad. Dementia is rubbish, isn't it? I too have bad days as well as good. I'll have a think,' I reassured him.

Now I prefer 'living as well as your circumstances allow' so people don't feel inadequate when they're struggling, and that is something that everyone can aim for, whatever their personal or financial situation. It's also open to interpretation because the idea of 'living well' for one person is not the same for another – and that goes for those of us living with a disease like dementia too. I know it doesn't trip off the tongue easily, or fit so well onto the PowerPoint slides that professionals are so fond of, but it's the truth. It comes with less pressure, less fear of failure, fewer impossible dreams to achieve. It is best for people with dementia, and isn't that what's most important?

ON BEING DISABLED BY OTHERS

We're at the local walk-in centre, as there were no appointments available with my GP. We've been kept waiting and inside my shoe my big toe thrums with pain. Sarah stands at the reception desk. A man sits behind the counter, tapping on a keyboard without looking up.

'I rang for my mum a few minutes ago,' she explains, until he makes eye contact with her. 'She has dementia and doesn't like using the phone.'

He casts his eye around the shape of her, to me standing there.

'What's her name, please?' he says, addressing Sarah.

She answers automatically, without thinking, but then the realisation dawns and she looks back at me, her eyes apologetic for not letting me speak. She stands aside a little so I arrive better into his view, a non-verbal exchange between the three of us.

'Date of birth?' the man says.

I clear my throat to speak, but as I open my mouth his stare has returned to Sarah. She looks at me. I tell him. Was that a look of surprise I just caught on his face? Or perhaps I'm being extra sensitive.

He turns back to Sarah. 'And what's the problem?' he says.

I wasn't wrong. I hear a sigh escape from my chest, but I'm too tired, and my foot's aching, and just this once I wonder if I've got the energy and patience to make myself known to him again. It turns out I haven't and so I nod my approval to Sarah, grateful that she's there and that she can explain quicker than I can. Once we see the nurse, I know I can take over from there.

So we wait on hard plastic benches alongside everyone else, and when we're called in, all goes well at first. I sit at the desk, opposite the nurse in her starched white uniform. She directs her questions at me, though I notice those split-second glances she makes towards Sarah, as if checking between sentences that I am telling the truth.

'Let's see this foot then,' she says, cheerfully, and as I lean down to take off my shoe, we almost clash heads. 'Oh, I was going to help you,' she says.

'I can take my own sock off, thank you,' I tell her, trying to keep any aggressive punctuation from my voice.

Her examination is completed with mumblings of, 'Getting worse before it'll get better,' and 'Should have come sooner.' Sarah, now a junior sister, joins her in their medical shorthand, so I let them speak for a while before I realise the consultation is over. The nurse turns back to me.

'Shall we put your socks back on again?' she says, talking to me as if I am a child, as if I need gentle and jovial persuasion, as if I am incapable.

I say nothing. Instead I pick up my sock and will my hands not to fumble just on this one occasion, as if I need to prove to her that I am perfectly capable of putting a sock and shoe back on. I'm annoyed when my fingers stumble, but it's done, and we rise to leave the room. But inside, I feel disabled somehow by the situation, by her language, her tone, her actions. I had arrived at the emergency medical centre a person of agency, yet their assumptions about whether a person with dementia can speak or indeed take off their own shoes and put them on again makes me feel less capable. Why do they group us all under one umbrella? Why do they treat us like children? Why do they focus on what we can't do, instead of what we might be able to? Why don't they see every patient as an individual person instead of a diagnosis when they walk in the door? Why does the medical profession rely on clichés and stereotypes and, as a result, so often gets it wrong?

ON DEPICTIONS OF DEMENTIA

Dementia is represented more often in arts and fiction these days, though accurate portrayals are not always found in books and television, and writers or screenwriters can often rely on clichés to get their message across to audiences quickly. Often these depictions focus on the very end stages of dementia or accelerated versions of the disease trajectory, forgetting that there is so much life to still be lived despite a diagnosis. It would be nice to see people in all different stages of a dementia diagnosis for the most accurate representation. But as the 2016 report says: 'Film and media producers do not merely set out to provide an accurate description of dementia. They have an interest in obtaining a certain impact, in providing entertainment,

suspense and dramatic effect. They allow themselves a certain artistic licence...'

This was certainly my experience when I was asked to
advise on the TV hospital drama series *Casualty*. Writers of
the show wanted to depict a storyline where Sister Duffy –
one of *Casualty*'s main characters – was living with dementia.
After the release of my memoir, producers reached out to
me, Dementia UK and my friend Suzy Webster, whose
mother was living with a dementia diagnosis, to name a
few. I first met with the story editors in London and, over
a cup of Yorkshire Tea, we discussed likely plots and plans
for inclusion. They took copious notes and asked me many
questions. They seemed very keen on researching the topic
thoroughly and wanted to get it right by listening and
learning. Only, when I started to receive the scripts, their
plans had apparently been derailed. Things had changed –
as happens in the world of television, I discovered – and
now there was a different team of writers who were taking
the storyline in a completely different direction from the
one that we had discussed. I didn't feel that the writers
were taking my suggestions into consideration any more
and were instead relying on the stereotypes that I was
determined to avoid. I decided that I couldn't work with
them any further because, for me, the depiction of Sister
Duffy's dementia needed to be accurate above anything
else – especially if I was going to be associated with the
storyline. I couldn't undo all my hard work advocating for
dementia if I allowed them to pin my name to the credits
of a show that had not taken my advice on board. I stepped
away, disappointed, but a few months later, the editor got
back in touch. There had been another change and this

time, she felt sure that I could influence the writers. When we met again, it felt different – better – a burning desire on their part to get it right. When the scripts started arriving, I could see that my thoughts and ideas had filtered through into the writing. I always knew they could never get it right for everyone because each person's experience of the disease is different – but they had to start somewhere.

When the show was aired, I couldn't watch all of it. Something about it didn't feel right, particularly the portrayal of someone with dementia, the little nuances of gesture and facial expressions. I wished that I had been able to meet the actress, to help her understand better. Sarah is an avid fan, and she'd often text me about bits where she could clearly see my influence, times when they had got it right, but they were few and far between. The ending was dramatic, but it felt designed to satisfy the appetite of the viewing public, to reaffirm what they already knew about dementia rather than break new ground. The last scene, if my memory serves me correctly, was of Duffy – having reverted back to her earlier days as a nurse wearing her original uniform – sitting outside in the cold, dying. I'm sure for the viewer it provided emotional resonance, confirming every stereotype they already had inside their heads. It is hard to challenge clichés and stereotypes; they are there because they work, particularly in a short TV drama, where they serve to speak in a shorthand to the viewer. But each of us has a responsibility that our portrayals of others are accurate, balanced and respectful, or at least that's what those of us with dementia ask.

News and media organisations still have a long way to go. How many times have you seen a news headline that describes someone living with dementia as a 'sufferer'? To address this, I worked with twenty of my friends at the Dementia Engagement and Empowerment Project (DEEP) on *Dementia Words Matter: Guidelines on Language About Dementia*. As people living with dementia, we know more than anyone how the language that people use to describe us not only affects society's view of us, but also the way we view ourselves. We produced these guidelines for journalists, organisations and communications departments when writing about or describing those of us with the disease. Words that should never be used, we concluded, were those that made us flinch upon hearing them. Words and phrases like: sufferer, demented, senile, burden, victim, plague, epidemic, enemy of humanity, living death. We recognised that particular words are used in headlines to 'catch a reader's attention' but asked that those words are not used in a sensationalist way, knowing that this just feeds stereotypes, clichés and negative images. This is important not just in terms of creating greater understanding within the population, but also so that those who may suspect they have the disease don't feel stigmatised by it and don't fear it. The more positivity that we can emphasise, the more that we can show people living with disease, the better for everyone – and that might even be the newspaper editors themselves one day.

ON COMMUNICATING WITHOUT LANGUAGE
Because of the societal stigma around a dementia diagnosis, some people do not want to make that diagnosis public. For them, language might not be appropriate, or available.

Some people do not want to have to explain the challenges they face every day, but with an invisible disability like dementia, it's not always easy to be understood in silence. For those times, I am grateful that there are visual signals that we can give people to let them know that we might need extra time, or even a guiding hand. Yet even the sunflower lanyard, which has become a symbol of recognition for all invisible disabilities, has caused a debate. The sunflower lanyard is an idea that was conceived in good faith at an airport so staff would be alerted to offer extra help to those who might need it. It spread outside of those departure lounges, into shops, government buildings, train stations and city streets. It is not just used for those of us who have dementia, but for anybody to indicate that they have a hidden disability and may need more time.

I would love to live in a society where I don't have to wear a lanyard to highlight that I might need help, where everyone is understood and there are no tuts behind me in the queue when I am taking a little longer with my shopping. But we are such a long way from that nirvana, and until we get there, something as simple as the sunflower lanyard will have to suffice. Not everyone is strong and confident, with the language skills to state their needs or their rights clearly. Some people need the confidence that wearing a lanyard gives them to go outside into the world and know that they will be understood that much better.

I travel up and down the UK extensively, trying my best to remain independent, and I know from first-hand experience that not all staff on train station platforms pick up on subtle clues of confusion or signs that someone is struggling. Sometimes, when I am wearing my lanyard, a smiley guard will approach me and ask if I need any help, even when things are going well. But the lanyard has come into its own on bad days – more often bad journeys which, if you use trains as regularly as me, you'll know are very often indeed. Journeys when trains are cancelled, when routes are changed at a moment's notice, make my brain feel ready to explode.

One such journey was on my way back from my paradise of Keswick. As usual it had been a lovely stay, but my journey home went from bad to worse. First, trains were cancelled. I stood on the platform feeling empty and lost, unable to work out a plan B, but then the sight of the ticket office caught my attention. I went over and simply asked what to do. The guard there was lovely. Once again, my sunflower lanyard came to my rescue – the guard glanced down at it, gave me a big smile, and printed me out two options with all the details of each journey. He assured me that I didn't have to worry and that someone would help me, and that smile and those words of comfort were all I needed to hear at that moment. The next challenge was the change of route, which meant that I would need to make an extra change, and that meant I wouldn't have a seat reservation, which I always relied on. Once I arrived at the unplanned station stop, I got myself a cup of tea and just sat on a bench, not quite knowing what to do. I must have looked totally lost when I got to the platform, as a guard came up to me asking if I was OK. I saw her eyes glance down at my sunflower lanyard, and just the sight of the yellow-and-green pattern completed the conversation for me. I said I didn't have a seat on the train and she told me exactly where to wait for a carriage that would have empty spaces. My journey could have been a disaster, but instead that subtle lanyard meant that complete strangers offered me help.

But there are some people who don't think that anyone should have to wear them; that if anything they disable us, or highlight our disability so that we might get taken advantage of. But we're not highlighting the fact we have dementia: we're communicating that we have a hidden disability, and for me the advantages still outweigh the downsides. In general, those of us living with dementia expose ourselves daily to others who can take advantage of us – especially people like me, who speak out about topics. Some also worry that by highlighting our disability we risk creating a two-tier system in society, which would single out people with dementia and prevent us from being able to blend in, leading to more judgement.

Of course, everyone has a choice whether to wear the lanyard or not, but people who do choose to wear them should not be made to feel bad about it if it makes them feel safer, more able to travel and better equipped to go out into their own community. As one friend said to me on Twitter when this debate was raging: 'It's an education tool – it can start conversations.' And as we have already established, conversations are the best way to change attitudes.

ON SOCIAL MEDIA

It is common for these types of debates to rage on Twitter, and as I've said before, putting your head above the parapet can be difficult. Conversation is not as easy as it once was for me, particularly a conversation that involves a large group of people, but social media makes that possible again. I remember when I first came across Twitter after my diagnosis. I simply sat, watching this silent world busy with communication and conversations that bounced back and forth between people from all different countries. Those in different time zones could sign in and take part in a debate; people living with dementia could share their experiences in different countries; we could figure out what was working where, and what we could do to bring it to where we lived.

Twitter was – and is – a place for us to swap ideas, to boost each other's morale, to provide support or perhaps just a laugh. It was a month before I even dared post my first tweet, but now I'm hooked. I can sit in perfect silence and have conversations with people I would never have met in my ordinary life. I've made friends, shared a lot and learned a lot. For someone like me, with a hidden disability, it provides a platform. It gives me a voice and it can change minds. In short, it grants people living with dementia – or any other minority – a place at the table.

I took part in some research with the University of Exeter. Researchers wanted to understand how those of us with dementia used Twitter and what identities we created and promoted for ourselves in this online world. My account was one of several that researchers analysed. Their findings overall indicated that Twitter was being used by me and my contemporaries to convey positive messages about the disease and for political lobbying for change and recognition of the need for inclusivity. 'Through their collective action, they are able to challenge traditional assumptions of dementia, have an impact on the practices and policies that affect their lives, and contribute to a greater social and political understanding of dementia,' the report says. It sounds great, but in reality, behind the scenes, I and many of my friends ask ourselves what is actually changing as a result of this. Progress can seem extremely slow and we don't have time on our side for all that red tape. What I do know is that those of us living with dementia on Twitter call our fellow followers our second family. We encourage others to join because we know there is safety in numbers. We look out for one another and we know that others look out for us too – especially when we're being criticised.

'Although Twitter advocacy work does not seem to be replacing offline advocacy, it is providing dementia advocates with an additional platform through which they can share their messages with a wider audience and challenge public perceptions of dementia,' the report says. We know that we can make a difference, but the reason this platform appeals to us is the brevity of the tweets, the limit of 140 characters. A long piece of text is impossible for me to read now, but a tweet is something that I can understand and engage with.

The report recognised that our collective work as dementia activists meant that we had caught the attention of the people who mattered – like politicians and lobbying groups.

This level of political engagement has not been evident for people with dementia on other social media platforms, which highlights the uniquely political nature of Twitter and is consistent with previous research showing that people with other chronic illnesses and members of the public use Twitter to influence policy-making and draw attention to social issues.

I often use Twitter as a way of getting my friends involved with research and, likewise, researchers now actively seek me out to promote their work and to gain participants, as my reach is usually larger than theirs.

The report discussed how those of us with dementia use the platform for the 'promotion of social movement', but the very fact that we can is often used against us. As outlined earlier in this section, there is a dark side – the people who question our diagnoses or troll us on social media platforms, accusing us of 'self-promoting' – but thankfully they are the minority, and if we really believe in freedom of speech then perhaps that is just something we have to accept. Twitter allows people living with dementia to connect, and connection is always going to be the best way of communicating with and educating people – *if* they want to learn.

I tend to focus on the positives of living with dementia, which was consistent with the researchers' findings:

The dominant narrative across all of the tweets analysed in this study is one of activism and living well. Other narratives, such as those of people who are struggling with their symptoms, were notably absent from the data ... It is possible that a lack of negative experiences being present in account holders' tweets could be an artefact of people who are living well with dementia, being those who choose, or are able, to interact on Twitter. This finding could also be due to account holders' use of Twitter to produce social change, where tweeting about the negative aspects of their lives could further perpetuate the stereotypes they are trying to challenge.

I do use Twitter to highlight the bad days too, as by not doing so we open ourselves up to more criticism that we are not showing all sides of dementia. It's also not fair on those whose bad days outnumber the good, because they may question themselves as to why they have so many bad days if the rest of us aren't being honest. I've also used Twitter as a helpdesk when I've needed guidance on my journeys. Once my daughters weren't available when a train was cancelled and so, in my panic, I took to Twitter and my lovely followers came back with suggestions that helped me to find my way home.

The University of Exeter report concludes that access to online communities such as Twitter not only provides those of us living with the disease with support, but that membership of social media platforms might 'help to reinstate a sense of identity among people with dementia, provide social connection, and potentially reduce feelings of isolation and loneliness that often follow a diagnosis'.

But to do this, technology firms need to be inclusive when building these sites, for example by making sure that navigating sites is easy for those with disabilities, and not having complicated security systems. Technology companies often consult with the public, but not people with dementia as a matter of course. Something as simple as a 'how-to' video, simple pictorial instructions or audio instructions would help people find their way around complicated web pages so much more easily. When creating sites for children, they make them simple and intuitive – why not for adults too?

Zoom has been another platform that allows me to keep in touch with my peers. Each week, we have a girls-only 'Zoomettes' meet from the comfort of our living rooms, which provides much comfort and support. Some of us aren't always in the mood to chat, but even those of us who are having a foggy day can log on and be ourselves in a community of others who know exactly what those bad days feel like. One friend of mine told me the other day that even when she feels too exhausted to take part and decides just to lie back and listen, she's soon laughing along with the rest of us, and that – for any disease – really is the best medicine.

ON TECHNOLOGY

As highlighted above, technology for people with dementia has to be fit for purpose and easy to use and set up, otherwise a good idea can quickly become a frustration. I remember my friend Agnes telling me how a firm had come along to set up a 'lifeline' for her husband, who has dementia, rattling off all the instructions he needed to know. But when they left five minutes later, he'd forgotten everything and was none the wiser about how to use this new technology he'd been given.

My iPad and iPhone are my door to the world now, my constant companions who never leave my side. My phone is instantly set when I have to remember something – the reminders are constantly pinging in my ear, some daily (like remembering to eat), some one-offs (like remembering to check on a friend who was feeling unwell). If something occurs to me that I need to do and I'm out for a walk, I simply set a reminder immediately in my phone for when I get home, otherwise the thought would be lost among my footsteps.

Technology has proved to be a godsend for my daughters too, who didn't have to worry where I was once they loaded a simple tracker onto my phone – it works both ways, telling me where I am too.

I've numerous apps that make life calmer and easier to navigate. For example, thanks to my train app, my love of travel has remained unhindered because it sends me alerts if my connection is delayed, and lets me know which platform I need to be on. My London Tube app tells me which station and line I need without me having to stare goggle-eyed at that wiggling map with all its different colours.

Alexa is another best friend of mine. She's there as a reminder to take my medication, and so much more than that – when I kept falling on the stairs, I discovered I could ask Alexa to switch the lights on upstairs by giving her a shout. I can even get her to boil the kettle for me, all from the comfort of my bed. I plod downstairs in the morning and can already hear the rumble of the element kicking into action. Like many other friends, we experience miscommunications too: sometimes Alexa doesn't understand my stammering commands if I ask her to switch the kettle on, and instead she's given me the weather forecast.

'I'll just do it myself, shall I?' I say, rolling my eyes.

To which she mutters something about not understanding and we go round in circles before someone gives up – usually me.

Many of my friends have Alexas too, and they all find it helpful to cope with life with dementia in tow. We have discovered, though, that's it's not too helpful when we're singing her praises on a Zoom call. One day, as we all sat around complimenting Alexa, her 'ears' pricked up at the sound of her name and suddenly chaos ensued as all our robots started chattering at once – mine even started to play Beethoven's Symphony No. 5.

There was much hilarity as we all started yelling 'Stop!' to our individual Alexas, and then fell about laughing. It is true that technology can be a blessing, as well as a curse.

ENVIRONMENT

If the sun is shining and I have nothing better to do, I can often walk for hours. It has not been unheard of for me to walk 28,000 steps around my village – or so my pedometer tells me. I have many routes that I take from my front door into the surrounding countryside, but none that take me too far from home— at least, I didn't think so.

I am often asked to try new products that those who are keen to tap in to the 'dementia market' think we might find helpful. I agree to try them on one condition: that I always write an honest review, and so it was like this that I found myself testing a new tracker watch.

The watch arrived looking very stylish and, sadly for me, very confusing. I asked Sarah to help me set it up, but even she got lost on the website it directed her to. Still, we persevered, especially as Sarah was to benefit too, as she would be the one tracking where the watch was placing me. She'd never had any trouble keeping tabs on me from the app we use on my phone, but we imagined this one would be even more detailed, even more accurate, and so I set off with it.

The text message came immediately: *What are you doing in Southampton, Mum?*

Eh? I'm in Birmingham, I texted back.

A glitch, we thought – a 150-mile hiccup.

Yet these mishaps continued. According to the watch, I was sighted in all sorts of places across the country as Sarah sat at home playing 'Where's Wendy?'

I decided to contact the company. They sent me a new watch and went to the trouble of setting it up for me 'in house' – not much use if you're a consumer, although Sarah and I were glad not to have to go through the rigmarole again.

So off I went on my travels once more, with Sarah watching my every move. Imagine then her surprise when I was spotted in Yangzhou, China. I've always wanted to go to China, but I'd never thought my bus pass would get me there, and I was in somewhere far less glamorous – Milton Keynes.

Sarah watched from home as I continued my Asian tour.

What are you doing in Japan?! she texted me a few weeks later.

I think that was when we knew it was time to give up. I'll stick to the lanes around my village – it's far less exotic, but at least I know my way home.

ON THE SEASONS

What can nature teach us about dealing with change? In times of struggle there are always lessons to be found in the world around us – even if that is only in our very own back garden. There is nothing that nature does not know about life and death, chaos and order, the light and the dark. I see it every morning and afternoon on the trundles I take around my village. I see that the waxing and waning of the seasons are necessary, that they stand as a reminder that there is nothing more natural than change, that it is not something to fear or avoid, to ask 'why me' when Mother Nature is so very undiscriminating to animals, plants and trees. Instead it is something to face head-on, to respect, to embrace. Sometimes, with this disease in tow, there are only the seasons that I have for company each day, reminding me that the small and incremental battles I win against dementia matter as much as a tiny acorn that falls from the tree and grows into an oak.

When I was diagnosed, it was July, but it may as well have been winter. I could only see the metaphorical leaves of my own tree stripped bare, that all awaited me was black nights and cold, still, monochrome days. I know some people stay there, in the darkness of their winter, resigned not to see the signs of spring after a diagnosis of a progressive illness. For animals, winter is a time for rest and recuperation, for hibernation, to conserve energy and recharge – perhaps that's what those same devastated people are doing as they retreat into themselves – I know I did for a while. But even now, in a world so frantic and busy, there are times within any day that remind me to rest and slow down and make life less complicated to give my brain a chance to recover.

When snow blankets the ground, there is beauty to be found in the simplicity of the world; for those of us living with dementia, an uncomplicated black-and-white land-scape is easier to navigate, much the same as it is for new-born babies. Trees stripped bare of leaves do not need to be seen as ugly if you take time to admire the beauty of their branches. Winter is a chance for me to spot the snowy owl swoop down at dusk from the paddock opposite my living-room window without the usual leaves that camouflage him. Just like the owl, the time limit imposed on those with a progressive illness means the necessity to find beauty in the most harsh of seasons, the most empty of places, in the now. Winter is a time to close the door, to snuggle in the warm, to rest and rejuvenate, something we all need to remember to do once in a while. Winter is a chance to turn the sound down on the world, just as the snow seems to do as it falls, to get back to the very basics.

In spring, I wait for new lambs to fill the fields that surround my village, or a nest of ducklings to take their few tentative paddles in the village pond. There is, of course, risk that comes with change – for those ducklings, it might be the heron watching from the rocks; for me, it might be a slippery pavement that my shoes fail to grip, a branch that springs back from the arms of a tree too soon and leaves me with a black eye. I could avoid these dangers altogether – I could stay inside with only this disease for company while I wait for sunnier days, but then I would be missing out on so much: the bluebells and crocuses, the daffodils that swarm the bank opposite my home. Spring is a reminder that there is always tomorrow, or next week, or next year. That a foggy day might be followed by a clearer one, that hope still flourishes after life changes, even if it looks a little different to the way it did before.

In spring, I fill boxes with seeds and plant them on my windowsills for the days when going outside might be impossible, when the fog comes down and blurs the world and the only respite from dementia is to curl up in my duvet and just watch the treetops sway outside my bedroom window. But even on those days there is hope in my seed tray, tiny green shoots sprouting, a reminder that nature will continue its course, that it will be waiting when I am ready to re-emerge. I think of these same seeds when I give my talks or write my books, hoping that the ideas I plant in people's minds will germinate, and that they will pollinate when people share them with others.

Nature is a part of our everyday language. People often use weather to describe their moods: dark clouds, crying rain, feeling sunny. Days spent in the sun are preferable to those spent under a cloud. But summer is a reminder that even when facing the sunlight, we tend to create a shadow. Nature knows you cannot have good days without the bad, that life – and living – is a perfect mixture of both. Plants need light and shade and water too. Just like humans. In the summer when I walk beside fields burned by the heat of the sun, I know we all need rainy days to replenish, to recharge and rejuvenate. Control over when they come and how frequent – as nature reminds us every day – is simply an illusion.

For me, summer is a state of being and not doing, especially on the days when the disease wins. You must respect nature. I remind myself of days sitting on Blackpool beach, toes stretched out in the sun, and in the distance the lifeboat crew responding to a call for help. The crew know that the sea's waves are too strong for most; they've learned to respect them through bitter experience; they work with the tide and not against it. It's the same for us when dealing with dementia. I choose to ride the wave because if I tried to fight it, I would only drown.

People fear the autumn, for what might follow, and yet it is filled with an abundance of colour and fruit. Autumn is about endings, yes. It is saying goodbye to a joyful summer, of late nights on the lawn, of the sun taking longer to sink behind our heads. Autumn is, by nature, a slow turning-out of the lights. Could there be a better seasonal representation of a disease like dementia? Yet to be fixed on what to come is, as I have said so many times before, a waste of all that nature offers us now – why focus on the winter when there is still an Indian summer to enjoy?

The burnt oranges and yellows of the last fading leaves on the trees; the miracle of plant life readying itself to survive a winter; animals and their instincts buried deep inside to plan for harsher times ahead. There is so much humans can learn from autumn about change and how to prepare for it, and when the leaves start falling from the trees, and I catch again that first glimpse of my snowy owl, I remember all that winter has to offer.

ON WALKING

Did I notice these seasonal changes before life forced dementia on me, reminding me I have nothing but this moment? My daily trundles are my moments of mindfulness; with a camera round my neck, I search my surroundings for something to capture on film – a moment that might be lost seconds later, if it were not for this digital memory.

I am lucky that I live in a village now, that I am surrounded by nature and all its beauty. I swapped town for country a year or two after I was diagnosed, when the sounds and hazards of the city became too much for me. What drew me to the house I live in now was the huge window in my living room, which overlooks the paddock across the road. I was fascinated that I was instinctively drawn to be closer to nature, as if I understood that on those bad days that would await me it would be my only company. But I am not alone. In a 2018 report, 'Overjoyed That I Can Go Outside', participants spoke about how being able to have a walk around their neighbourhood gave them not only a sense of freedom and empowerment, but also made them feel that they were keeping their own disease at bay. Walking definitely gives me a purpose, and having a purpose keeps my brain working. I don't walk aimlessly; I'm always looking around to see what I can see. It's the social contact as well, the navigating of the walk: all of it serves to keep my brain active. I can't walk with someone and take photographs – I can either walk with someone, or walk on my own taking pictures. Even if I am walking with someone, I tend to keep stopping if we're talking, as I can only do one thing at a time.

In the 2018 report, participants talk about what nature means to them, many of them admitting that, like me, the changing of the season gives them purpose: 'Maintaining a connection to nature was felt to be restorative and the participants shared their excitement at spotting animals or the pleasure of looking at flowers during their day-to-day movements through the neighbourhood.' Pre-dementia, I loved walking and seeing beautiful scenery, but it was all about distance then: how far I could walk rather than the detail of what was around me. Now I take the same lanes and paths every time and never get fed up, seeing something different each day: the first snowdrops in the village; the patterns the clouds make; the changing colour of the sky. Just like me, it seems that the participants of the study get so much pleasure from nature: 'The changing seasons symbolised hope and the chance to rejuvenate for some of the participants as they began to notice the early signs of spring after a long winter,' the report says. 'Time spent outdoors in nature was combined with restorative practices such as walking that helped participants to manage life with dementia.'

There has been a lot of focus on the habit of those with dementia to 'wander'. It always surprises me that it's only people with dementia who are 'wanderers'. Before their diagnosis, they might just be known as 'walkers'. People with dementia have a purpose, even though it may not be obvious to others. Walking might be the only thing they can do that preserves the little autonomy they have, as the participants in the 2018 study explained:

Earlier studies have suggested that people with dementia experience a shrinking world following diagnosis, often as a result of the progression of dementia, however our findings differ from this conclusion ... We argue that people with dementia actively challenge the prospect of a shrinking world by exercising a freedom of movement ... Such learning is of value as it provides a counter-narrative to earlier studies that have tended to pathologise the movement of people with dementia, especially those in the latter stages of the condition, by labelling it as 'wandering'.

The environment that we live in goes hand-in-hand with how readily available a daily walk is. The report goes on:

People sought out green and open spaces that were free of traffic and crowds which allowed them to move more freely without facing the stress or challenge of busy roads or congested pavements ... Walking through the neighbourhood enabled freedom of movement, something that reinforced a sense of autonomy, allowing people to feel in control of their lives, and at times to escape the pressure of isolation associated with their home life.

ON MAKING PLACES DEMENTIA-FRIENDLY

A World Health Organization (WHO) study, focusing not on dementia but on ageing in general, pinpointed people's desire to feel part of a community. 'Social participation and social support are strongly connected to good health and well-being throughout life,' the *Global Age-Friendly Cities* guide reported.

> ... older people consulted by WHO indicate clearly that the capacity to participate in formal and informal social life depends not only on the offer of activities, but also on having adequate access to transportation and facilities and on getting information about activities ... An age-friendly city emphasises enablement rather than disablement; it is friendly for all ages, not just 'elder-friendly'.

It goes on: 'Empowerment and self-worth are reinforced in a culture that recognises, respects and includes older people.' As I have always said, get it right for people with dementia and you get it right for everyone.

Transportation is also an important factor. I remember how a change in a bus timetable left all of us villagers discombobulated until we got used to the new timings. For somebody with dementia, that can potentially be a huge challenge to face.

The report went on to highlight practical things that make neighbourhood environments age-friendly. These included public seating, toilet facilities, dropped kerbs, ramps to buildings, adequate signage and safely timed lights at pedestrian crossings. The lack of any of these things might make the difference between someone going outside to enjoy their local neighbourhood or not.

But the most important thing in my opinion is people – people who understand what dementia is, and want to make the environment inclusive to us.

Here's how people around the world are getting it right, according to a 2017 report on dementia-friendly communities by Alzheimer's Disease International:

- The Netherlands started dementia cafés in 1997 and now has more than 230 of them, with 35,000 unique visitors. Organisations there also created DemenTalent, which aims to build on the talents of people living with dementia, offering them voluntary roles within their communities based on their abilities.
- In Austria, Aktion Demenz created 'memory parcours' so that walkers in local parks can gain information about dementia 'on the go'.
- Taiwan launched Dementia-Friendly Stores in 2013 to encourage shop owners to become more dementia-

friendly and enable people living with the disease to continue doing their own shopping. This includes advance payments, easy returns for unwanted items, and alerts to family when the person with dementia has been in so they know they are safe.

- South Korea has developed a 'dementia simulator' to educate young people about what it might feel like to live with dementia. Nursery-school children spend time in care homes, and schoolchildren are trained to give hand massages to care-home residents.

- In Japan, Kizunaya helps find work opportunities for people with young-onset dementia, including making use of vacant fields to start growing mandarin oranges for commercial sale.

- In China, the Yellow Bracelet Project was initiated in 2012 to encourage safety and prevent people with dementia getting lost. It has now become a symbol of affection across the nation. Safe Bracelets have now been launched, which feature a GPS tracker and have reunited almost one hundred people with their families.

- Alzheimer's Australia conducted a study in 2014 to discover what changes could be made in physical environments that would improve access and inter-action in communities for people with dementia. The report outlined suggestions such as minimising noise where possible, fewer reflective surfaces such as glass, and better maps, signage and directional cues.

When the new shopping centre in Leeds opened, I was so excited to pay it a visit. The flagship store was John Lewis, and I was instantly transported to the one I used to go to with my mother when I was little. It had a restaurant inside, and all the staff dressed in old-fashioned black waitress uniforms, their frilly white hats matching their starched aprons, serving tea in china cups and saucers out of a shiny silver teapot. It may as well have been tea at the Ritz for me as a small child.

Gemma drove me there one day, and we arrived at the large gleaming building with automatically opening doors. But it was then that I came to an abrupt halt. Gemma charged in, yet I stood stock-still. The marble floor was a polished black ocean of grey swirls that looked like waves. My head was already spinning and I felt nauseous before I'd even taken a step inside. Gemma looked round and saw me static at the door.

'The floor looks like water,' I said, and she took my arm as I managed my first tentative step inside. As we walked along, I had to stare straight up at the ceiling to avoid feeling sick, trusting Gemma to guide us to our destination and hopefully away from this horrible floor. I'm sure it looks aesthetically pleasing to many, but for me – and others with dementia – it is a total nightmare to navigate. It seems such a simple thing that architects and interior-design specialists could be aware of to make the experience so much more inclusive. It didn't stop me going on that occasion, but it would fill me with dread for future visits.

I have been asked many times for my opinion on buildings that are meant to be designed to be dementia-friendly, and I'm always so surprised by the small changes they can make that would make a huge difference. As the

2020 World Alzheimer Report says: 'Good design is no more expensive than bad design, and there are substantial operational and quality of life benefits to be gained from it.'

Back in 2016, I was asked to look around a new building at East Riding Community Hospital in Beverley, Yorkshire, which hospital managers had hoped to make inclusive for those of us with dementia. After all, many of us would be using this local hospital. The team that I was assessing it with broke into pairs so that we wouldn't be influenced by one another as we wandered around the building, but we all encountered similar problems. The glass on the main doors looked very swish, but as it was tinted, you couldn't see inside and that just made the hospital look closed. Signage was the biggest problem: many signs were in a silver colour pinned to a pale background, which all blends into one for someone with dementia. Bright blue signs with bold white writing worked much better. Mostly it was the blandness of the place and the lack of colour: everything was beige, every door closed, many of them the exact same colour as the walls, without bright signs to signal who or what was on the other side of them. Something as simple as artwork from a local school would cheer the place up, or signage on the floors in different colours, depending on which part of the hospital you needed to get to, would help. These things wouldn't cost much, yet they would make all the difference to someone with dementia visiting the hospital. The problem is that we are often invited in to give our opinion once everything has opened, when it can be more costly to put things right. People with dementia need to be involved at the design stage.

The 2018 report 'Overjoyed That I Can Go Outside' mentioned earlier in this section highlighted the importance of places to sit for people with dementia. 'Benches had an important role to play beyond providing respite during a walk; they facilitated more opportunistic forms of social engagement and encouraged people to venture out of their homes as a result.' I can't walk as far as I used to, but we have lots of benches scattered around the village, so I always know there's somewhere to sit. When I'm there, people seem more likely to come and chat, just like the report said, or to see if I'm all right. One villager came out of her house to see if I was OK when I was sitting on the bench opposite her window.

I remember once going to visit a hospital to help the managers find ways to make it more dementia-friendly. They had installed some brilliant artwork in the corridors, which was wonderful, but there was nowhere to sit and admire it. I suggested some benches opposite.

My local town is very small, but one year the council decided to build a shopping centre just a short walk away from the main parade and they had the genius idea of putting large circles on the pavement to point the way both to the new shops and to the train station. Those of us with dementia often walk looking down, just because we don't feel so confident about where our feet might be going, so this worked really well.

One GP surgery I visited scored many Brownie points with me for its use of colour to define different areas, but lost points for the big staircase, which often moves in the vision of people living with dementia, and the swirly, decorative carpet that looked alive in the reception areas. But as I told them, friendly staff and big smiles make up for a lot. Martin Quirke and colleagues wrote about this in a report on dementia-enabling neighbourhoods. He wrote that 'a socially supportive environment can help to compensate for a less supportive physical environment'. It would be nice to work towards getting both things right, the physical and the social, but humans really can make the biggest difference.

ON THE NEIGHBOURHOOD

Where you live is of huge importance when you are living with dementia. I don't think people pay enough attention to the trauma of moving when you have a disease like dementia in tow. They think, like I did, that a move will just go like it's always gone. I got lucky in the environment that I picked because my village gives me access to lots of green open spaces for these invaluable trundles of mine. My three-bedroom house was perhaps not the best decision, though; it's too big for me to rattle around inside alone. Some friends of mine moved from their house to a flat, thinking that it would be better, but the noise from the homes coming through the floors and walls around them was so disorientating that they had to ask the council to move them to a bungalow. But when choosing a new environment post-dementia diagnosis, it's worth considering the access that you'll have to outdoor spaces and transportation, and what's on the other side of your windows. I never close my curtains – I feel isolated and alone if I do, trapped inside – so they're always open and neighbours will wave at me as they pass.

The 2019 Cambridge University Press report high-lighted the importance of windows that look out at neigh-bours and make people feel a part of their community, even if they are inside, and also how we get to know the daily sights and sounds of our neighbourhood.

This study underlines the importance of understanding neighbourhoods 'in time', as their character and features alter during the twenty-four-hour period. Many of the people we spoke to commented on how it felt when a quiet atmosphere descended upon their local area, sometimes as a result of being left behind when others went off to work or school during the day. Other studies have found that windows were sources of informal interactions and a sense of belonging by getting a smile through the window for older people with limited mobility and for people living with dementia … just to hear voices or see children playing outside gave hope and a sense of connection.

The routine of daily activity outside is comforting to me and sits alongside my own routine in harmony: the car doors shutting, engines starting as neighbours leave for work, the chattering of schoolchildren as they make their way to lessons, the horses' hooves clip-clopping on the tarmac roads, climbing the hill towards their field to exercise, the riders waving if I'm in view. Everything is orderly and in its place for the day, and it all happens again at the end of the day, but in reverse; that routine, that consistency is important. It's a reason for me why the school holidays disturb the equilibrium: it feels as if there is something missing and throws out my own routine. The report revealed others felt the same:

> For many people a quiet neighbourhood atmosphere was experienced as anything other than relaxing or peaceful, participants discussed feelings of insecurity during times when there were no people in sight. This underlined how just seeing people outside provided a degree of neighbourhood connection but also perhaps how it deeply reinformed a sense of neighbourhood identity.

Animals are more reliable; they don't change their schedules like us humans. When I'm upstairs in my bedroom during the day, the squirrels and the birds in the treetops are my companions, scurrying from branch to branch, chasing one another round and round the tree trunk.

I always wave to villagers if I'm out for a walk and see people at their window, just in case that's what they're looking for: that validation that they exist and have been seen by someone. If I need to be alone but outside in the fresh air, I'll go out at dawn to see the sunrise, just to feel the comfort of nature's routine. The sun never fails to rise and fall, giving me some structure to my day.

My home is my safe haven, especially when it's a bad day. The garden or even the view of a garden through a window can be very calming. I love sitting in my sun room and just watching the birds feed and the plants grow. You may feel numb inside some days but the view shows you life, just like my little seed trays on the windowsill

I feel lucky that I can still walk with the aid of my flexi stick. Taking those steps makes me feel normal, just like everyone else. Not everyone in my village knew I had dementia in the beginning. They knew me as the 'camera lady' because I would take photographs of animals or plants or fields around the village and post them on our Facebook page. Being the 'camera lady' made me feel good, because they saw me as a person, not 'a person with dementia'.

I asked some of my friends how they found navigating their neighbourhood these days. People have very mixed experiences:

'It's my Alzheimer's that stops me going out on my own. I used to; I went all over the place. But now I don't have any sense of direction at all. I go out one way and then I can't remember which way I'm supposed to come back. Apart from being in my garden, I don't feel very secure in myself. I did get lost one day and I wasn't a million miles from home, but it was the panic that set in.'

'I can go to the shops on my own, but yesterday I went to the shops and I felt so frightened coming back and thought, "Oh, I'm not going out on my own any more." I think it might have been a one-off and I'm going to have to fight it. If I get in a pickle I'll ask for help, and people have brought me home before. I went to the shop yesterday and I sat on a bench for a rest. This teenager came up to me and asked if I was all right, and I said: "Yes, I'm just having a rest." He asked if I was going to the shop and I said yes and he said: "Come on then, I'll walk with you." It was so lovely.'

'I go around every morning. I get up quite early and go for a walk on my own around the town. It's a very established regular walk. It's a simple time to walk around.'

His wife said: 'I've got Find my Friends app, so as long as Bob has his phone in his pocket and switched on, it makes me feel safer that he won't get lost.'

'I go out on my own, go into town, no problem. My daughter got me a phone for my birthday and she's putting a tracker on it, as I do get confused sometimes, but I'm perfectly all right. I don't mind asking people for help.'

ON FEELING LOST

The fields that I walk in around the village where I live are as familiar to me as my own footprints. I could walk that route with my eyes closed – although that might not be such a good idea, given the fight I had with a branch the other day that left me with a black eye. But twice a day I pass by those fields, and I know every curvature of their boundaries. To me, those fields are beautiful at every time of the year. There is always something to stop to take a photograph of as I make my daily rounds: a golden sunrise, a pheasant, or a robin come to keep me company. I feel safe in those fields, surrounded by villagers who know me, who are taking the same route, enjoying seeing nature do its work in all seasons, come rain or shine. We share cheery hellos and comments about that very same weather. And between their smiles, I stand alone and click on my camera shutter and capture these fields that I know so well, amazed all over again at the green shoots that spring from the black earth, keeping secret underneath them the potatoes that are growing.

Yet one day, as I made to continue on my trundle, I looked up from my viewfinder to discover that I was in a place I didn't know at all. I was still in a field, yes, but not the one that I knew. This field had no markings to identify it as one of mine; none of the usual familiarity was apparent to me. There was a pathway, one that I had come from, another that lay far in front of me, but I had no idea which way was which. I scanned the field for people, for landmarks, and found myself totally alone. That's when my heart started to race inside, the panic mounting alongside the questions. If I kept on walking, I knew I would be lost.

Don't panic, I said inside. If I waited long enough, I knew that a villager would appear, someone who could show me the right way home. So I walked slowly, trying to take my mind off the utter disorientation of the moment by viewing the world through the body of my camera, clicking away in the hope of growing calm. That's when I spotted them: two figures coming towards me, a man and a woman, a bright red coat. My heart calmed to a more comfortable rhythm. I smiled as they came towards me, and they returned the gesture with two of their own.

'Is this the way back to the village?' I asked, pointing up the path in the hope that my internal compass might just have set me on the right course.

'Hello, Wendy,' the man said, 'that's it, just turn right at the end of the path and you'll be there in no time.'

Turn right, I told myself. That was the answer I needed. I thanked them and continued on my way, repeating it over and over, and snapping photos as I went. Moments later, I was there at the end of the field and as I turned right, just as I had been told, the world suddenly came into sharp focus. Of course I knew where I was. There was the edge of the farmer's field, thoughtfully planted full of wild flowers, and his house with the black dog sitting beside the gate; there was the big oak tree on the right, and the path back towards home.

I picked up my camera and viewed the scene through its lens. Of course I knew this place. For today...

ON LIVING AT HOME

I have spoken many times of my insistence that I should stay at home and live my life independently for as long as it is possible. I know I am not the only person who feels that way. What we need to hear from our friends, relatives and professionals is not what is not possible, but how it can be made possible. As architect and design pioneer Margaret Calkins – who specialises in designing builds for those with dementia – said, her light-bulb moment came when she realised 'that the predominant deficit thinking about dementia had to be replaced with strength-based thinking, if the human rights of this growing group of individuals were going to be respected and supported in society'. I have often talked about how professionals should focus on what we *can* do, rather than what we can't, and that applies to all areas of our lives, including our homes and houses.

In her 2020 report, Ash Osborne talks about the import-ance of keeping things as they have been within the house for as long as possible to 'enable the person with dementia to enjoy their relationship with their past life, as embodied in their home, despite the problems introduced to their life by dementia'.

It is true that it's all of those things around us that tell the story of our lives. I only need to look at my brightly coloured bowl of shells to cast my mind back to days spent on Blackpool beach: instantly I can conjure up the sound of the waves, or the feel of the surf lapping between my toes. For that reason, these items are not to be seen as clutter or surplus to requirements, even if they are not deemed important by others. These things are the touchstones of my life. Often, people who move into care have such small rooms to live in that they have to discard so many of these items, which must make them so sad.

Osborne's report lists some ways that modifications can be made in somebody's home to help them live better with dementia. This might be making structural changes to the house, such as widening doors or corridors, or removing a wall to make the living area more open-plan. It is important for somebody with dementia to be able to see both where they are going and where they have come from. When I first moved into my own home, I would often get disorientated by a closed door once I'd moved from room to room, forgetting what was on the other side of it once I had traversed through. My answer was to take a screwdriver to those doors and remove them. That way, when I was in the kitchen, I could see through to the living room and vice versa.

Non-structural changes to fixtures and fittings such as ramps or grab rails can also make a huge difference for people living with dementia at home, particularly if they are prone to trips or falls. It gives them confidence to move about their house. But it's important to remember that although safety is of course important, your house is first and foremost a home, and many of my own friends have commented on the importance of the house not being made to feel too clinical just to put the minds of our loved ones at rest.

There are fairly minor changes that can be made in a home to make it more dementia-friendly. Swirly patterned carpets must go and be replaced with contrasting tones. Lighting is another important adaption that can be made. In my experience, I'm afraid to say, the energy-saving light bulbs are not very helpful to those with dementia, simply because they take such a long time to brighten – by the time you can see clearly inside the room, you might have forgotten why you're there at all.

Osborne's report continues:

> a number of researchers in this area have suggested that home modifications are best completed in the early stages of dementia, at which time they can have positive effects on the levels of confusion and support successful ageing in place. Modifications attended later in the disease process may cause confusion and impact negatively on the person living with dementia.

It is true that it is best to try and foresee problems before they arise in order to get used to the changes while it's still possible. Even decorating a room in a different colour from that which it has always been can lead to confusion and a feeling that a room isn't someone's own any more.

Decluttering is a simple way of creating a more relaxed environment for somebody living with dementia: removing hazards that can cause people to trip, like rugs or slippers, and small pieces of furniture like occasional tables or footstools. I don't like untidy clutter on my worktops, but then I like things on view to know that they exist – like my iPad or phone, keys, pen and paper, or timers in the kitchen. The only things that I put away are clothes and crockery, or food in my cupboards – but even in that case, I have photographs I pin to the doors to know what's behind them. Some people even swap wooden kitchen cupboard fronts for glass ones to enable themselves to look and see what's inside. Here are some ways that my friends cope with life at home with dementia:

> 'We've got more organised. I always leave my keys, glasses and handbag in one place now, as they used to be all over the place, but now they're in the same place each night and, remarkably, still there in the morning. The key is organisation, really.'
>
> 'On my drawers and wardrobes I've got a little list saying pyjamas and thermals and so on, so I know what's inside. But Alexa is our main thing: she reminds us of everything, when to switch the heating off, when to turn the lights out, all sorts. So I've got two women in charge of me now!'

Adjusting the living space so that you can look out of a window can be an invaluable way of adapting a home. I talked above of my joy of looking out of the window, of seeing life go by, of waving to people and seeing them wave back. Ash Osborne's report remarks on the 'significant effect on their sense of connection to their neighbourhood' something as simple as a window to look out of can achieve.

Noise is a factor that must be taken into consideration. It has been said that noise for people with dementia is what stairs are for people in wheelchairs, and so the less auditory stimulation, or rather interference, the better. It's the reason I have put my washing machine in the conservatory, so that I can close the door and not listen to its rumble when it's on spin. However, it does play a lovely tune when it's finished to tell me it needs emptying – that isn't so painful to my ears. There's a house in my village that has an air-conditioning machine attached to it and it disturbs me so much that I avoid going down that lane since they've had it installed. It's incredible what can be so ordinary for one person, yet so intrusive for others. Carpets and curtains can be a great way for absorbing sound, unlike laminate floors and wooden blinds.

ON MY MEMORY ROOM

My memory room brings me instant calm and warmth whenever I step through the door. I rarely just sit here, saving it instead for those days when I need to feel connected to my life, to be reminded of all those smiling faces staring back at me, all the images of places that I have stood, where I have pressed down on the shutter of my camera. This is just the spare room upstairs in my house, but it is so much more than that. It is filled with so many photographs of happy memories and says as much about

me as the blood running through my veins – especially on
the bad days when I lose my grasp of who I really am.

In front of me, at the top of the wall, is a red string of
photos held in place by tiny coloured pegs. These are of
the young Sarah and Gemma, and as I look at them I feel
the smile arrive on my own face. One in particular catches
my eye: Sarah, around eleven, and Gemma eight. I can't
remember where it was taken, but they're both looking
over their shoulder, smiling at me, the happiness written
bright across their faces. Moments like that captured on
film are worth their weight in gold. I'm reminded in a
second how well I knew every expression on those two
small faces; the joy, the embarrassment, the 'go away Mum,
I'm not in the mood for photos'. I turn slowly in my room
and, with each photograph, memories come flooding back.
There are photographs too of my happy places: Keswick
mostly, but there's Lulworth Cove and Durdle Door, and
one lone seagull silhouetted against a Blackpool coastline. I realise then that most of the photos involve water of
some type – a beach, a lake, a village pond. Something has
always drawn me to water.

In the corner, my memory boxes are stacked three high
now. I started with only one, filling it with my girls' first
shoes, but perhaps the panic of forgetting makes me more
inclined to save even the smallest thing now.

As I said, this is just a room inside my home, but it is so
much more than that. It is the present that brings me here,
but it is from the past that it has been created, a tapestry of
my life, and all its wonderful people and places. One foot
inside this room grants me my history. In a second I can
feel like a child again, or a new mother, a single mum, or

a proud one when I glance at my girls' graduation photos.
I feel calm in here. I remember who I am, and I don't need
to close the door to keep dementia out. This is my sanctuary; here the disease doesn't exist.

ON HOMES AND CARE HOMES

It's understandable that families like to have a sense of
security when their loved one is still living at home, but
they must remember that they wouldn't want to live in
a prison – so why would someone who has dementia?
There can be a tendency to double-lock doors and put
measures in place that would make someone feel that they
are trapped. This is mostly done with the best intentions,
but in truth only makes a carer feel more secure.

A 2020 University of Liverpool report focused on how
the right physical structure of a care home can have a huge
impact on the well-being of the residents. It warned against
visible security measures. 'Residents living in facilities with
camouflaged exits and silent electronic locks had lower
levels of depression,' the report's authors wrote. 'Overall
the benefits of security measures must be balanced against
potential harms of people with dementia feeling they are
segregated or restrained in a secure environment.'

One solution I have heard repeatedly is placing a curtain over the front door if somebody is prone to leaving
the house. If a curtain is there, it doesn't look like a door
that needs to be explored, but if it had lots of locks on it,
it could make you feel as if you were trapped. This also
goes for access to the great outdoors in care homes. The
same report talked of how beneficial it is to people with

dementia who have access to gardens and other outdoor areas and so 'restricting access ... may have unintended consequences'. One of my friends recently moved into a care home and she can only go outside if a member of staff is there to accompany her. This just makes her feel trapped and closed in, and it has led her to be very depressed. Surely, if there is a garden attached to a care home, it should be easy to access and safe to wander around as a matter of course – or the architects of the place would have to ask themselves why it was so badly designed. Residential homes that feature therapeutic gardens, which include memory boxes, wandering paths, scented plants and viewing platforms where residents can watch wild-life, report not only improvement in quality of life, but reduced agitation and depression in residents, and also less stress for staff and family members.

Of course it's important for care homes to focus on creating the best environment for residents, but their friends and family should not be forgotten either. The University of Liverpool report said: 'In small-scale settings family members have reported being treated more as group members rather than visitors and were able to join at mealtimes. This encouraged family members to visit their relatives more frequently.' It is good to hear that this is being addressed: often there can be so many rules at care homes, which deter rather than encourage visiting. I remember one family I met who told me: 'Mum's safe now – she's being looked after, so we don't need to worry. They'll ring us if she's ill.' But they never visited her because they couldn't bear to see her in a care-home environment. Stories like that make me feel so sad.

ON DEMENTIA VILLAGES

For me, the jury is still out when it comes to 'dementia villages'. De Hogeweyk in the Netherlands has been hugely lauded, and is the inspiration for many others cropping up around the world – the Belong villages in the north-west of England have a similar approach. The De Hogeweyk model is a gated village close to Amsterdam that is home to 152 people living with dementia in its twenty-three houses. The size of ten football fields, the village has its own town square, theatre, garden and post office, where residents live seemingly 'normal' lives, residing in groups of six or seven to a home. They are, predominantly, for people with severe dementia, but the idea of segregating any demographic of our population always concerns me. Residents are cared for by 250 staff who are specialists in dementia, but they also hold down jobs within the village, such as in the shops and grocery stores. The restaurant and the pub within the village are open, not only to residents but their friends and families and the staff who provide care for them. It sounds good in theory, and apparently the average client-satisfaction score for De Hogeweyt was 9.1 compared with a countrywide average of 7.5 in regular care homes, but there is something about them that feels so unnatural.

I had a dream the other night that I was taken through these high steel gates, controlled by someone I couldn't see and, once inside, they clanged shut behind me. I instantly felt trapped, like I was a prisoner here to serve time until death took me to a nicer place. As I walked those streets inside my dream, everything felt like a pretence. There was crazy laughter, as though people were mocking those of us with dementia who were staring into fake shop windows with fake goods never to be sold. There was lots of colour, but no soul. I tried a door, but the handle didn't even turn. Inside this nightmare everybody walked in twos except for one man who passed us, whispering in my ear, 'I'm escaping,' as he shuffled along a circular path that would never set him free. I wanted to leave but, like all the others, I had reached that stage where I was no longer capable of being heard. The new me gave in, and with that feeling, I woke with a start, so relieved to find myself in my own bed that just for confirmation of the fact, I asked Alexa to switch on the lights.

I have to be clear that this was just a dream, but it is obvious what my subconscious has to say about such places. I'm sure they are wonderful for some people, and these stylised environments for people with dementia seem to be becoming increasingly popular. Glenner Town Square outside San Diego claims to 'break the mould' of what a respite centre looks like. This 'village' is contained within a warehouse on the edge of the city. Once inside the main lobby, visitors are met with what looks like an old 1950s theatre, a small diner set with tables to eat at, a pub with a pool table, an old car at a petrol station, a barber-shop, a 'department store', a mini museum and even a cinema that seats twenty people. Personally, I don't like these fabricated, unnatural environments, but I can see how they would be stimulating to some. For me it would feel confusing to have a car sitting at a fake petrol station that never moves. I once visited a cinema room in a care home, and it was all black and felt completely disorien-tating. What worries me about these places is the thought process behind them: is it the people they aim to serve, or the companies who come up with these novelty ideas to make money? I don't like the idea of people capitalising on any disease.

I do, however, think that respite care can be a good stepping stone for people who want to explore moving into residential care, or just a day's break for someone who is living with dementia, or the person who cares for them. One of my friends, Chris, looks forward to his days in respite care, simply because it is a rest. He can sit in silence all day if he wants, whereas at home he perhaps feels he needs to be available for conversation. His wife took a little more convincing, as for her it felt as if she was 'sending him away'. But that doesn't have to be the case, and it can be a welcome break for both people.

In Norway, one model that has worked is 'green care', where traditional farms are opened up to community members with dementia. This is better than a fake environment in my opinion, and just as stimulating. In these facilities, those living with the disease can help in the kitchens or gardens, chop wood, pick fruit from the orchards, eat together and go for walks while their regular caregiver gets some respite. The Norwegian national Dementia Plan believes 'environments must not only compensate for functional decline but build on a person's own resources and strengths', which I am thoroughly in favour of.

EMOTIONS

True friendship does not grace us as often in our lives as we would like to think. It is something that is beyond any description. How can I accurately describe my closest friend in these pages? A whole lifetime of knowing her would not be able to do her justice in words.

I met Sylvia when I was thirty-nine. A single mother to two young girls back then, I'd made ends meet for years with various cleaning jobs. Like many people, I was trying to avoid acknowledging a deep sense that I could do more with my life if only I were brave enough to risk failure. The job advert for a receptionist in a hospital physiotherapy department would be the push I needed. I circled it, then left it at first – there is more safety in what we know. But that job advert wouldn't just mean a sharp handbrake turn for me, and the start of a career in the NHS that would last almost twenty years – it would lead me to the best friend in all the world.

As the office manager, Sylvia sat in on my interview. Apparently the head of the department was unsure whether to give this single mum a chance, but Sylvia persuaded her that my status would only make me more reliable – I needed this job, after all. Her instincts served her well. I was first to arrive and last to leave. It was the stepping stone that I required, and Sylvia took my hand to guide me.

I was used to being alone, protective of my independence. Yet there was something about Sylvia that I could trust. We were different in many ways – she was outgoing; I was deeply private – and in other ways similar. We were both fiercely loyal, we did not suffer fools, and we both had two daughters that we adored. We were almost the same age, though she reminded me constantly about the 'almost'. A year younger than me, she teased me that I tried all the major milestones before her. She wasn't keen on forty, despite my assurances that it had gifted me the new beginnings that the number promised, so on her big day I covered the windows of our department with huge letters that the girls had helped me colour in, reading: *Look Who's 40 Today*. I watched her approach from the car park, her forehead creased in confusion as she spelled out each letter and then the eye roll and her trademark smile as she found a photograph of herself pinned to the door and realised instantly who was behind it. From that day we became firm friends.

We were to each other the sister that neither of us had ever had. We both liked to keep fit, and so I taught her tennis, not realising I had unleashed a monster who became determined to beat me every time we stepped onto the court. That serious frown of concentration as she waited patiently, tennis racket in hand, swaying – just as I'd taught her – from foot to foot as she anticipated my serve, became another one of our jokes. Sylvia hated the thought of getting wrinkles, so I'd tease her whenever that famous frown appeared and she'd instantly swap it for a smile. Our trips to Wimbledon became a favourite, picnics packed and Centre Court tickets in hand. I have kept every single one of them in my memory boxes.

When her first husband left her, there was no need for words, just that one plea for me to come over. We sat in the living room of her quiet cul-de-sac semi, her two Westies on her lap and me bringing tea from the kitchen. Often in our friendship we didn't need to speak to know what the other was thinking. A few weeks after her separation, I persuaded Sylvia that she needed a change, so I revamped her bedroom with my famous decorating skills as she watched on, 'supervising'. Many a bottle of wine got us through those days. There were highlights too, like the holidays in the Lake District that Sylvia introduced me to. We'd climb to the top of Walla Crag and sit with just the breeze for company before I guided us back down – a sense of direction not being one of Sylvia's strengths.

We celebrated the happier moments in our lives too. When Sylvia met David she was like a teenager again, and dragged me along for a weekend in Keswick to test if she missed being away from him. We decided to fill our days with long walks, and Sylvia bought a set of walking poles just like mine. The only thing was that she was much shorter than me and oh, how we laughed at the sight of her walking along with these two giant sticks. We paused along the Keswick Railway Footpath to try to work out how to shorten them, but no matter how we tugged and twisted, pushed and pulled, nothing happened, and soon we were helpless with laughter. We saw an elderly lady approaching, a stern look on her face, and when she got near, she snatched them out of our hands, adjusted them and went on her way – all without saying a word. We stared after her, not daring for our eyes to meet until she was well out of earshot, and then we howled with laughter.

When I was diagnosed with dementia, Sylvia was determined to learn everything that she could, but as my best friend, it was the change in my emotions that she noticed the most. She understood better than anyone how my range shortened to register only happiness, sadness and contentment. There were no sliding scales for me any more, as if my brain had to power down its scope to concentrate on more vital things at hand. Unlike most, Sylvia got it, and the bits she didn't understand, she asked until she did. I shared my research with her, and she was always interested, curious with ideas. So when she was diagnosed with ovarian cancer some years later, she tackled her own challenge in just the same way. It was research that kept Sylvia alive for years; she tried new drugs and learned everything about new treatments.

Throughout all of those ups and downs, we still met up a few times a year. Only one day, I felt a necessity to see her, just sensing inside that something was wrong. I went by train for the day and, true enough, she'd received bad news from her consultant.

'I didn't want to tell you because I knew it would make you sad,' she said.

In that moment, if I could have taken the cancer from her body and installed it in mine, I would have done. Sylvia still had so much life to live, whereas dementia had already claimed my future. I would have happily taken the cancer from her so she could have spent more time with David. But it was an impossible dream.

As the cancer took hold and all treatment had been exhausted, she was admitted to hospital, but once again, she didn't tell me just how bad things were. She didn't have to: I felt it. It was coming up to Christmas, my favourite time of the year, and she was determined that her own dimming spirit should not spoil mine. Right up until the end she was thinking of others.

Sylvia was allowed home for the last few weeks, to spend the last of her days, hours and minutes with her husband and daughters. A hospital bed was installed downstairs, and afraid again to tell me the truth, she instead consulted Sarah on whether she should let me know she was about to die. Thank goodness Sarah persuaded her to, because I wouldn't have missed those last few beautiful conversations we shared for anything. It's a strange thing when you have dementia and you know that your best friend is dying. It wasn't me so much I was worried for, but others – what if, when the time came, I forgot Sylvia had died and sent her a message? I hated the thought of upsetting David. It's bad enough living with this disease myself, but I didn't want it to cause pain to others.

As Sylvia grew weaker, our messages stopped. At least we had said everything we wanted to say. One winter's morning, I received one simple – yet beautiful – text from David, which read: *A very bright light went out at 03.05.*

Always bright in our hearts, David, I wrote back.

David told me that Sylvia's final wish had been to hire a caravan to come and see me. They'd even worked out how to keep the electricity running for the machine she was hooked up to, but it was never to happen.

I have often talked about the two bookcases in which we hold our memories when we live with dementia. There is the factual one, the one that is flimsy and rocks from side to side with this disease, sending the books tumbling onto the wrong shelves – mixing up memories and years and people. But there is the more sturdy one that stands beside it, and that is our emotional bookcase. Perhaps I had forgotten that nothing rocks that. It is the place for the memories that have meant the most; the shelves for those we have loved the deepest, who have made us happiest and the loss of whom we feel deeply. I know now that that is where Sylvia is sitting, and there, on the shelf, that bright light will never fade. I didn't need to worry about forgetting her death when there, on that bookcase, she is alive within me.

There are some days when the sadness has overwhelmed me, when even a trundle through the village cannot pull me from my grief. I know what it felt like to feel sad before dementia, how one sad moment could send you into a spin, opening up the memory of other difficult moments like some kind of sadistic Russian doll. But it is not like that now. It is as if this disease, which can be so cruel in so many ways, doesn't allow me to dwell too long on those saddest of moments. Sure enough, soon another scene flickers into my mind when I think of Sylvia's death – a walk up Walla Crag, a game of tennis in the sunshine, a glass of wine in her cosy living room.

Sylvia knew my love of robins and how I believe them to be the spirits of those who are long gone. The night that she died, I had the most wonderful dream. In it, I asked Sylvia to come back to me as a robin, and give me a sign that she was still with me. In my dream, a new robin appeared in my garden and I went outside, hand held aloft with seeds and pieces of suet. The robin flew over, gently landing on my hand. It took a tiny seed, looked up at me and held my gaze, and then promptly pooed into the crease of my palm. I laughed so hard, yet the robin didn't move. I knew then: there she was, my best friend, come to say hello.

ON OUR ABILITY TO FEEL EMOTIONS

It is not unusual for those of us who live with dementia to have a different experience of our emotions after diagnosis. It is hard to pin down how much of this is caused by the disease itself and how much might be influenced by the medication that we are prescribed in the hope that it might slow the progression of dementia. There is very little research in this area, as I discovered during the writing of this section, and the only thing that I can put this down to are the assumptions that are long held by society – even professionals and academics – about the emotional life of those of us who have been diagnosed with a disease in our brains. The problem is, as I have said many times before, that once we received a diagnosis, people stop seeing the human and instead only see the disease. It is a mistake that is made over and over again, yet it can feel to us as if little is being done to address it.

A scan of research papers on the subject of the changing emotions of people living with dementia reveals very little at all. Almost all literature is about the carer's emotional experience, even though we are the ones living with the disease, and it strikes me that if people tried a little better to understand our emotional selves, there might be less talk of 'challenging behaviour'. We might just feel a little better understood.

I consulted my friend Dr Jan Oyebode, professor of dementia care at Bradford University. 'When it comes to formal research, the missing part is research that has set out specifically to understand the emotional experience of people living with dementia,' she explained. 'I would still say that in my several decades of clinical contact with people living with dementia, that dementia does not affect people's ability to experience a full range of human emotions, but it manifests differently for everyone. We all know from our contact with people living with quite severe dementia that people may have trouble speaking, remembering and so on, but we still see people being happy, sad, angry, frustrated, contented and showing all the emotions any of us would.'

In fact, rather than an assumption that the emotional life of someone living with dementia is surplus to requirements, emotions can actually be key in preserving the sense of self, because they give a window through which to return to past memories. In her 1997 paper, Marie Mills's research concluded that 'emotions associated with their past experiences appeared to provide a strong cue to recall and formed a significant feature of their accounts as well as providing all informants with narrative identity'. I can relate to that, with just a wander into my memory room. I definitely find that memories in my life with the greater emotional pull hold tighter to my grey matter. I can still conjure up the sadness I felt when I was attending a talk in London and was forgotten as a speaker. I had been all ready to go on stage, prepared notes in hand, and they just didn't announce me – they skipped me altogether for the next speaker. I was so devastated to be overlooked.

We often talk about neuroplasticity, where our brain may be damaged in one place but uses another route to enable us to do or remember things. If the motorway is closed, we use the B roads, and that's what our brain does too, even in someone with dementia.

The Mills report concluded that:

> the characteristics of emotion and duration of memories, which are associated with autobiographical memory, imply a relationship between emotion and available long-term memories in older people with dementia. Moreover, a certain strength and durability is indicated in the emotional autobiographical memories of informants that was not apparent in other aspects of memory.

It went on, 'memory appeared to decline more quickly than the emotions and the emotional responses of informants'.

Another study aimed to explore the full emotional spectrum of being diagnosed with young-onset dementia. A 2017 report by Charlotte Berry found that four emotions were most prominent: fear, anger, sadness and contentment.

> The findings indicated that participants experienced feelings of fear and vulnerability in response to their diagnosis. Participants felt angry that they did not have a voice, not enough was being done for those with dementia and they were being stereotyped. Participants spoke of a more depressive state of mind in which they grieved for their past self, experienced isolation and loneliness, and feelings of hopelessness and despair. Finally, participants spoke of a sense of contentment

in relation to a preserved self, a sense of living alongside their dementia and a desire to live in the present;
making the most of the here and now.

I asked some of my friends what their experience
had been:

'Since diagnosis no one asks how do I feel? What are
my thoughts? I feel stripped of everything, of being a
person, a mother, a grandmother; only by meeting peers
did I find my voice. I take medication, and I wonder, did
I only find my voice because of that? When I see others
being treated like they haven't got any feelings by services, I speak up for them because I remember how
I felt after my own diagnosis.'

'My doctor has never asked or allowed me to talk
about how I'm feeling, or if I do query some of the
changes that are happening, it is as if he doesn't want
me to go into detail. Everything is: "Oh, it's just your
dementia." Yet my neurologist says: "Well, it could be
your dementia, or something else..." Nothing is ever
discussed in depth or detail. Some family members
don't even mention my dementia; it is as if they are
scared to talk about it.'

'Researchers are not interested in emotions; they're
interested in what they can do to make things better,
but equally there is a misconception – a huge one – that
people with middle-to-later-stage dementia, who look
quiet and calm and don't say anything or perhaps can't
communicate verbally, are brain-dead, but we know
from our limited early experience that actually there's

loads going on even if I don't express it. I don't see why
that would stop if you simply lose the function of putting your thoughts into words.'

I believe that we are emotionally functional right through
to the end, it's just – as my friend just said – people can't
see it, but it's visible if you look carefully enough. I often
think that professionals are almost embarrassed to talk to
us about the emotional side of our lives because they don't
have the answers for us, and if my research is anything to go
by, it's because nobody is asking the right questions. I know
that my emotions are still there after being diagnosed with
dementia, but they do manifest in different ways.

ON SADNESS

A few days after Sylvia died, I was with Sarah, and I was
conscious of us talking about something sad, and then
a moment later me suddenly being happy. The same
happened when I was walking with a friend: I was telling
her about losing Sylvia and that made her sad, yet just when
she wanted to ask more questions, I skipped to something
happier and felt fine again. It must seem very strange to
other people, but for me, with this new way of thinking, it
somehow feels normal.

Many people I know have died since I was diagnosed and
yes, I've felt sad. But Sylvia was the first person I lost who
I was very close to, and the sadness was difficult to cope
with, but I haven't cried as much as I thought as I would.
I found myself wiping my eyes when I was writing my
blogposts about her, and I certainly did when I received

the news of her death from her husband and when her daughter contacted me. But the tears don't hang around for long. Dementia has given me the ability to have short-lived moments of grief, followed quickly by extreme highs of happy memories.

Curious to know more, I asked my friends how their experience of sadness had changed for them. While all their responses were different, it does confirm that, like me, their relationship generally with emotion has changed since their dementia diagnosis. Here's what they had to say:

'For me, sadness has changed quite dramatically. I find that if something sad happens to me, I could cry for days over it; it sticks in my mind and lasts longer than happiness does. Only the other day, I was walking down the street with my husband and a funeral car came past us, and out of the blue I just started crying. My husband said: 'What's the matter?' And I said: 'It's just so sad, there's a person there that's dead.' I wouldn't have done that normally. Everyone knows it's sad to see something like that, but it's like my emotions have become heightened.'

'I do find that I have periods: five minutes, an hour, a whole day, where I'm just overwhelmed by sadness and I don't know what about. I feel like crying and have tears welling up. If you're sad, you're sad about something that's happened, but the instant weeping and emotion feels entirely different. You imagine yourself unconsciously to be in the position of the person who is describing it and that chokes you, and you just can't stop yourself from being in their head in that moment.'

'I don't feel sadness any more. I am more emotional and I do get weepy over things that would never have bothered me before. I cry at the drop of a hat. But I don't feel sadness like I once did; for me there is a difference between sadness and weeping. I'm more sad for other people than myself, but then again, I've always been like that. The empathy is still there.'

ON FEAR

Empathy seems to be heightened for all of us with dementia. Yet there is a common misconception that those of us living with dementia don't feel empathy like we once did. In 2016 researchers from Neuroscience Research Australia studied people living with Alzheimer's and behavioural variant frontotemporal dementia, more commonly known as Pick's disease. This particular dementia has become better known, thanks to the work of comedian and writer David Baddiel, whose father lives with the disease. The study concluded that people living with Alzheimer's and behavioural variant frontotemporal dementia had a reduced capacity to understand and appreciate the emotions of others, known as cognitive empathy, although this could also be as a consequence of general cognitive decline. But in the group of people with behavioural variant frontotemporal dementia, there was a significant difference in how they were able to share the emotions and emotional experiences of others, known as affective empathy. Neuroimaging revealed that the loss of empathy in these participants was due to 'Pick bodies' in the part of the brain that is integral to social functioning.

Unfortunately, though, when this research was reported, the headline was often 'dementia causes loss of empathy' and that is where many misconceptions stem from. People forget there are more than one hundred different types of dementia. You would never lump together all people who have cancer, and the same should go for those living with a complicated brain disease. Among myself and my friends, although none of the people I interviewed have Pick's disease, all of us still report high levels of empathy for others. In fact, what we most often find is that our sadness related to ourselves has diminished or disappeared, perhaps as a result of accepting that we have no control over the future.

This loss of control over the future is often seen as a negative by those of us living with dementia, and it definitely contributed towards a feeling of fear for many of us when we were diagnosed. As I have discussed before, that fear for me was perpetuated by the negative images, languages and perceptions of life with dementia. My first real experience of dementia was my own diagnosis, and so I didn't have any other images to combat the view that society had fed me. Such is the fear of dementia that there have been studies on 'dementia worry' which, according to a 2012 study is the 'emotional response to the perceived threat of developing dementia'. The report cites a 2008 British survey by the Alzheimer's Research Trust that found that dementia was second only to cancer among the most feared diseases:

Overall, 26 per cent of the respondents reported that they were more afraid of dementia than of any other condition. Among respondents over the age of 55, dementia was the most feared condition, with 39 per cent of the respondents reporting that they were most afraid of dementia, and 30 per cent reporting that they were most afraid of cancer.

Because of society's image of dementia, it obviously perpetuates that fear, just as the word 'cancer' struck the same fear into people years ago. While cancer is still feared, people know that you can still lead your life with the disease in tow, and that treatment is increasingly successful. Many cures are available simply because of the amount of money piled into research, but this has been lacking with dementia – hence the image of it remaining stuck in time. It seems to us living with the disease as if Alzheimer's charities have decided to focus more on care than cure. Pharmaceutical companies have been trying for years to find that elusive cure, but I expect that the breakthrough discovery is more likely to target the start of the disease – perhaps even twenty years before symptoms start showing – when drugs can be brought in to reverse the progression while dementia is still a seed.

The report continues that people tend to have an 'overly pessimistic' view on living with dementia:

In a sample of 186 Jewish and Arab adults with no family history of Alzheimer's disease, the mean hypothetical emotional stress that participants expected to experience if they were to develop Alzheimer's disease was 4.0 on a five-point scale ... Significant proportions of a large sample of third-generation Australians (27 per cent) and Australians with Italian (54 per cent), Greek

(60 per cent) and Chinese (46 per cent) backgrounds indicated that people with dementia no longer enjoy life.

These perceptions explain why those of us first facing a diagnosis felt so terrified of an uncertain future. The fact that there is even a phenomenon known as 'dementia worry' tells us that we are talking about living with the disease in the wrong way. The report goes on to talk about how, with every life-threatening condition,

[a] moderate level of worry/fear arousal is thought to be optimal for engagement in health behaviours such as screening: whereas too little fear leads to denial and lack of attention and too much fear may lead to avoidance, as people are too afraid to have their fears confirmed. In line with this assumption, multiple studies suggest that a moderate degree of cancer worry is the most conducive for motivating cancer screening behaviours.

The report's authors question whether this would also translate to dementia worry, but unfortunately, so little is known about the disease that it is impossible to know how to avoid it, except for maintaining a healthy life with a good diet and regular exercise – although that was how I lived my life pre-dementia.

The report discusses how there is a 'negativity bias' towards the quality of life for those of us living with dementia. It is why so many of us try to share our lives through blogs and social-media platforms: we feel that if we can dispel some of the myths, it might mean that a positive diagnosis has less of a negative impact.

I asked some of my friends how their own relationship with fear had changed since their own diagnoses:

'When I was a child, I was fearful of everything; I never wanted to do anything because there was always a danger. But that's gone now. I can't think of anything I'm frightened of.'

'I don't fear for my future. I used to – at the beginning of my dementia I felt fear. I felt fear that my life was taken over by other people. But as I've gone along, I don't let them. I don't fear the future; the only fear I do feel is ending up in a care home. That's my only fear, but I have made a care plan; whether it gets carried out, I don't know. I don't want to go into a care home; I don't want that total loss of control.'

'I don't think I'm more or less afraid of anything. I don't feel fear about anything, except perhaps losing confidence and how I would cope if something went wrong if I was ten miles from the house.'

I still remember what fear feels like: those heart-pounding moments, frozen to the spot, my legs weakening under the pressure of making the next move – fight or flight. What brought on those momentary sweats then? It seems ridiculous now, but most likely it was a dog coming into sight. That sudden feeling of the hairs on the back of my neck prickling to attention, my blood tingling with adrenalin. I love dogs now, but back then I would cross the street to avoid being within yards of one – now I do the opposite and cross the street to meet them. Those fears seem irrational now, but they were very real to me then, haunted by the memory of a black dog in my childhood chasing me as I pedalled for my life – or at least that's what it had felt like at the time.

I don't remember when it happened, but I remember the sensation of that fear melting away. It felt like a relief, to let go of this emotion, to free up space and allow animals into my life. What was it about dementia that took this burden off my shoulders? I have always said that it was facing the fear of my own diagnosis, that nothing could be worse than that for many of us, as the statistics from the dementia worry report confirm. But I am not sure it was only that.

I had the same fear of the dark, another thing that stemmed from my childhood and stayed within me my entire adult life. I'd rush to put the lights on when I arrived home on a winter's evening. Now I step inside and forget, wandering around, sometimes stumbling in the darkness but never considering to put the light on to guide me. I get pleasure from staring at the blackness outside my window, the midnight sky, the moon, the stars twinkling back through the glass. My curtains are always open now. But back then, they would have been tightly shut, my house inside lit up like a Christmas tree. Even being out in the dark was something to be avoided; the fear of an attack always lingered in the back of my mind, my brain conjuring up all sorts of stories as to who might be waiting for me in the shadows. Now it's for different reasons that I sometimes avoid the dark: dementia creates different shadows that appear as confusing apparitions; the tones of pavements and roads blend into one, which mean that I stumble often. But sometimes my need to see the moon overrides this, and I tolerate the confusion just to lay my eyes on its steady and reliable permanence.

ON ANXIETY

Fear and anxiety might seem intertwined in some way – perhaps we get anxious about the things we fear the most. But without that fear, there seems to be less to be anxious about. Now what my friends and I worry about is having control taken away from us. We fear being taken out of our own homes and put into a care home. We fear falling over the edge. But it's a very human thing to worry about the loss of self. The same dementia worry paper I mentioned above addressed this issue:

> ... unlike other fatal diseases, dementia not only threatens the physical self but also aspects of the 'symbolic self', the very aspect of human identity that separates humans from other animals. Terror-management theory argues that people have a need to distinguish themselves from animals and seek a higher and more meaningful existence ... In Western culture, cognitive capacities, autonomy and internal control are central aspects of the symbolic self. Qualitative studies on the experience of dementia have revealed that both healthy participants, as well as people with dementia, emphasise the themes of loss of independence, identity and control, as opposed to more physical aspects of dementia. Dementia thus seems to threaten the very idea of individuals' identity as human beings.

Time is usually the trigger that makes me most anxious. If I'm due to be somewhere, or perhaps plan to attend a Zoom call online, and yet I haven't received an invitation and I can see the clock ticking towards the allotted meeting time, that makes my head spin. Before it would just annoy me if people were late – it was their problem, not mine. I was always on time. But now the anxiety about time can feel quite overwhelming. I hate going for GP appointments because my doctor always runs late. I try and keep calm in her waiting room, telling myself that it's because she cares so much about her patients that she always spends the time that is required on them, but something overrides my logic. I see the clock hands go past the time of my appointment and then irrational thoughts flood my brain: has she forgotten about me? Has she missed that I am here waiting? Did I remember to book the appointment? I'm exactly the same when a taxi arrives late, immediately fearing that I forgot to book it, or that they have forgotten about me. I suppose that says more about my lack of confidence in myself, because I don't have the memory to rely on that I did check and double-check something in the same way others might. I also might forget I'm meant to be waiting for something, and go and start something else instead.

I can cope when I know something is going to be delayed, for example if a guard at a station tells me the train will be eight minutes late. It's when they don't have an answer, or the dreaded 'delayed' sign appears on the information board with no clue of its arrival time – or if indeed it will ever arrive – that I begin to feel anxious. My village bus used to cause the same anxiety in me. Again, it would be because I doubted myself: had I got confused and missed it? But since the bus company introduced a tracking app, I am much calmer.

Again, with the lack of research on dementia and anxiety, I surveyed my friends to see what their experience was:

'I don't get anxious any more over things. I am more agitated, and I'm less patient than I was with myself. I've got loads of patience for everybody else, but not with myself. If I'm doing something and it doesn't go right, I get very cross, whereas before I would keep calm.'

'I'm more on an even keel now. I don't know whether it's since I got the diagnosis or giving up work, so I therefore don't have the anxieties associated with that. I've always had an intense lack of confidence; I used to worry so much all the time what people were thinking. When I was driving along, or walking along the pavement, I was always scanning, wondering, "Are people looking at me? Are people saying something? Is it about me?" I couldn't live my life very well, but I know that anxiety and lack of confidence is childhood stuff. But that's calmed down now. I do feel quite happy with my life as it is. I feel at ease with my life, if only because I have put all those other aspirations and fears and all that "I can change the world" stuff into a bin somewhere. That's the past now; that ain't going to happen. It's difficult to accept that, but I think it's an important part of why our feelings settle a bit when we have dementia. We no longer have that pressure of a future on us. I care less about what I should care about; if it's not in my heart or head, it's not happening. So I'm not going to put myself out to pretend it is.'

'I used to worry and try to fix things for everybody before, but I don't tend to worry about anything now. I get anxious about it, but I think, "I can't do anything about it now," so I tend not to try and fix things for others. I had a bad accident before my dementia – I got hit by a car – and from then I learned things were out of my control. I do worry about my family, but I don't worry about life or myself. I don't worry about my future, whereas I used to before.'

What my friends say resonates with me too. Dementia has taught us that some things are out of our control, and that anxiety won't be able to do anything about it.

ON ANGER

There are some changes to the ways I experience my emotions now that I feel must be down to the disease itself and the changes it has made to my physical make-up. Since my diagnosis, I have always pictured the inside of my brain like a network of road systems: there are flyovers and motorways, roundabouts, junctions and, of course, dead ends. What dementia has done to this highly complicated system is add in several roadworks. It means that my thoughts have to take diversions, some fast, mostly slow, and sometimes they just don't reach their destination at all. Out of the billions of cells that make up my transport network, there are perhaps only a few thousand that are affected by dementia – the reason I can still do many things myself – but it can be so frustrating if one of the places I want to travel in my brain is disrupted by these roadworks. More and more, as the disease progresses, I am noticing more diversions and dead ends, and one of the things affected is my emotions. I know the destinations still exist in my brain – I can still happily make it through to sadness and happiness without any hold-ups whatsoever – but other places are seemingly unreachable to me now, whatever clever diversion I might attempt to come up with to outwit it.

There was a situation a few months ago where I knew I should feel angry. Those of us living with dementia have complained for so long about the lack of services to help us at the point of diagnosis, people who would be able to show us that it is still possible to live with dementia. Our frustration with clinicians reached such a stage that my friends and I from my Minds and Voices group decided that we would write a course ourselves that would be delivered by those of us with dementia for people newly diagnosed, to help them understand what it was really like to live with the disease. We wanted to give them some hope, instead of that dismissal after diagnosis that there was 'nothing that could be done'. We called our course 'A Good Life With Dementia'. It would be six weeks of emotional and practical support with no abandonment at the end because each person, if they so wished, would be able to come and join our regular group.

We managed to get funding from the Clinical Commissioning Groups and were supported by the local county council to run the course. Only we quickly realised that it wasn't being supported by clinicians. No referrals were being made by the very people who were the gatekeepers to the newly diagnosed, even though we were ready to help them. I knew I was meant to be angry. My initial thoughts set off down what was once a familiar path to the department marked 'anger' in my brain. But I just couldn't get there. It was as if that emotion was encased in a steel box. It was completely impenetrable to me. Instead my mind immediately set off down a more familiar route, one that had a better chance of reaching its destination – and so I arrived at sadness. I knew there was something missing in me, some wholeness, that range of emotions that make me human. I wanted to be angry, I felt I *should* be angry. But I just couldn't be.

The same system of roadworks can sometimes work in my favour too. I see other people get angry and realise that this use of their energy is fruitless, that the outcome is impossible to change, that they will only cause themselves more grief by feeding the anger inside them. But it frustrates me when I know that something could be changed if only I could channel my anger into something productive. The truth is, it is just not there for me any more.

I wondered if some of my friends who live with dementia had the same experience as me:

'I don't get angry now, I get more frustrated. Anger seems to have gone completely. I'm quite calm now. My husband gets angry over things and I say, "There's no point in getting angry – just forget it." But that's how it is now. I can't see the point in getting angry over something, whereas before I would have done.'

'I get angry about things at the drop of a hat – silly things. I have always been short-tempered, but it's the more trivial things now that tend to trigger it. For example, I have a zip on one of my fleece pullovers, and it's taken to not working, and I try and pull the thing up and it won't go, and I do it again and again, but on the third time I get quite close to ripping it off. I cannot control that as well as I might have done in the past.'

Perhaps, as with all of these things, a lot depends on our personality before dementia, though I for one know I used to rant and rave and feel that adrenalin running through my veins. But is that feeling one to miss, or in this case has dementia done me a favour? Most of the time I'm relieved that anger is now inaccessible to me. It makes for a far more simple life. When you have dementia you need everything to be clear-cut and simple: we embrace the black and white that life has to offer, as the grey nuances are just confusing to us. To know I'll be happy, sad or content is fine by me – most of the time.

ON GUILT
Guilt is something that often feels as if it goes hand in hand with a diagnosis of dementia. How strange when people are most used to feeling guilty if we've deliberately done something wrong. There is only one type of dementia that I know of, Wernicke–Korsakoff syndrome, where you could possibly say that someone contributed to their own failing health, as it is alcohol-related. But even then, it was as a consequence of behaviour – it wasn't something people actively sought. So why then does guilt play such a large part in our lives?

My first experience of it was at the point of diagnosis: that rush of guilt for my daughters, that I had somehow robbed us all of a future together — even though I knew I had simply been unlucky. Up until that point, the three of us lived happily independent of one another, each getting on with our own adventures. I was Mum, I offered a listening ear, a place of refuge when things went wrong, but other than that I was happy that my girls were getting on with their lives — as I was getting on with mine. The guilt came when my mind flashed forward. Images of being unable to help them in the future flooded my mind, pictures of them caring for me rather than the other way around.

Unlike many people, I had no guilt for my immediate future. I had no partner at home who had to live alongside me or make adaptions to help me cope with this new disease that had invaded our life. It helped that I had no shared dreams with someone to shatter. I've since heard from so many friends of mine who talk suddenly about the 'burden' that they become on their husband or wife, forgetting that we are no different the day after our diagnosis than we were the day before. The partnership is still there: it will just have different challenges to face. But then, doesn't that eventually happen in every marriage? Dementia can feel as if those challenges come to meet us sooner than we had thought. I saw partners who, like me, had projected themselves into a future that no longer existed; instead of reminding themselves of the mantra that there is life with dementia, their minds were bombarded with images of the 'trip of a lifetime' they would now never take, or exciting plans for retirement that would now be swapped for something altogether more sedate. I know that it's in those times, when those pictures flash into our minds, that the guilt arrives: it reminds you of what you've taken away from others. Because that's how it feels; it's not so much what you've lost, but how this disease will impact those who you love.

I have witnessed it for myself: the husband who wishes he could still take his wife a cup of tea in bed in the morning, but once he arrives in the kitchen he has no idea what the process is any longer and needs his wife to help him. There are these everyday losses to deal with as well as the bigger picture. I feel I am lucky not to experience that. My other single friends agree. 'If I forget something, I forget it, it doesn't matter to anyone else,' one told me.

I have met people who have made their partner feel bad about all the things they're not able to do, yet for every one of those people, I know there are those who would never consider describing the person they love as a 'burden'. One couple I remember meeting recently talked to me about this very subject. The man, who had been diagnosed, spoke about the tragedy of not being able to change his situation, but said: 'I can't help having dementia, that's what's so cruel.' He talked about how he didn't want to put his lovely wife in the position, as he described it, of being 'man and woman of the house'. Yet she insisted, 'Our marriage vows said in sickness and in health; we just take one day at a time.'

One couple who I am friends with explained to me how guilt affects their relationship. Bob, who lives with dementia, spoke of his contentment knowing that his wife, Sue, would be there to pick up the pieces, but that in itself made him feel guilty that his disease had put that pressure on her. 'That's not the way round it's meant to be,' he told me. Sue, on the other hand, said that having to do things has 'made me more confident about how things work and how to fix things as Bob's confidence wanes'. She has come to see the very thing he feels guilty about as a positive. Another friend talked about how she feels guilty that she was always the homemaker and now her husband has to take over those roles in the house.

I remember feeling my guilt more acutely at the beginning. One friend, more recently diagnosed, said her feelings were centred on her role as wife and mother, and in her case, grandmother:

'The guilt side of things for me at the moment is quite bad. Everything I do or say, I feel guilty because I have dementia. I feel I'm putting something onto my husband; it's something we didn't plan for and I can't get that out of my head sometimes. I suppose for me it was more the guilt that this is my second marriage and we've only been married about fourteen years, so it's a relatively new marriage. I felt the guilt that he could have married anyone but he married me and now I've got dementia, and he's now going to be looking after me. But he always says he wouldn't have it any other way. I feel very guilty that I can't help my children out like I used to with the grandchildren, and that is something that eats away at me, and then the sadness comes. The guilt for me at the moment is awful.'

ON HAPPINESS
There's another type of guilt that I have become accustomed to, and that is the guilt of happiness. It sounds

strange, but sometimes, in this world that dementia offers me – stripped of the same pressures that others are under; an escape from the hamster wheel of life that people are still desperately spinning on – my contentment in the moment, my ability to find the best that this disease has to offer, makes me feel guilty. I have been living with dementia for many years now, and, as I have said so many times, my glass half-full approach is one of the ways that I might appear to cope better than others. But I know for other people it is not so easy. I have learned how to find pleasure in the smallest of things. When I return home and log on to Twitter, seeing the tragedy of the world outside of my own on some days – of man-made disasters or cruelty, or simply reading the thoughts of others who are struggling with their disease that day – I feel guilty for the happiness that I have found for myself. I wish then, in those moments, that I could give some of it away. I can see that my positive outlook must really annoy those who are having a difficult day. That, for me, is a strange kind of guilt to feel.

But would I even describe happiness in the same way as I did pre-dementia? The happiness I saw for my future when I was sitting in my office at work, wishing the days away until the weekend, or perhaps even retirement, has certainly changed. For me, happiness comes in smaller packages now. I was never materialistic; I didn't dream of objects, big cars or big houses. However, I might have dreamt of exotic holidays, or a run along the coast at night-time. I had dreams of travelling the world, visiting far-flung countries. Of course, I've had to let those drift off into the ether. So what makes me happy now? A day when my head feels calm; or seeing a bird singing away to its friend; being out for a trundle, capturing a squirrel peering out from the trunk of a tree. I've learned to see the beauty in tiny moments now, rather than a bigger picture that somehow always left me wanting more.

I feel excitement at the prospect of a visit to Keswick, but that always settles quickly into contentment. Happiness, or excitement, is more like a butterfly that flutters around on a summer's day in the garden, impossible to pin down. Yet contentment feels like something we can hold in the palm of our hand and examine, taking more pleasure with every glance. Even my beloved trips to Keswick are riddled with concerns about the taxi arriving, or the train being on time. Yet nothing spoils the contentment of the moment when I finally reach the lake shore and sit on my favourite bench looking out across the undulating fells.

I wondered if my friends' relationship with happiness had changed since their diagnosis:

'I don't feel happy, that emotion of happiness is gone, but I have more joy, more contentment. I get more enjoyment out of things, like my allotment. I'm more content with my life. I have more time now to just go outside. I stop more and listen and look around than I used to. That's joyful to me.'

'Simple things make me happy now, whereas before I was quite materialistic. I always had to have a sports car; now that does not cross my mind one bit. It's the same things now, like walking on a beach – if you took that away from me, I would be devastated. And my crafting gives me pleasure too. I can get lost in the moment of the crafting. I've done something for me that I've wanted to do, and I've enjoyed doing it. Everything I enjoy doing now is surrounded by nature, getting out and doing things.'

As you can see, happiness for me, and many of my friends, involves mindfulness of the moment, an appreciation of the present because, after all, the past can often be a blur and the future is a complete unknown. But then, has anything really changed? Shouldn't all of us live in the moment more? It's just that we got out of practice. Think of how much pleasure a toddler has in examining a tiny shell on the beach – nothing will distract her from her task. Yet as we get older, we get out of the habit of focusing on one thing; instead we let desire for other things spoil the moment that we have in front of us. We focus on the lack, rather than what we have. More than anything, dementia has taught me that we all need to return to the moment at hand.

Charlotte Berry's 2017 report on young-onset dementia looked at this same idea of contentment in the present moment:

One of the experiences that participants spoke enthusiastically about related to the value of a time in which dementia did not exist and during which they became fully immersed in the present moment. It is possible that the experience that participants came to value as important to them could be understood in the context of a state of 'flow'.

Apparently, 'flow' occurs when people are absolutely absorbed in a task, which is what my friend above talked about with regards to her crafting or me when I'm taking photographs. In that moment, she doesn't feel that dementia exists because she is so focused on the task in front of her. The report states: 'For participants, the ability to maintain concentration on the present moment and reduce self-consciousness meant that they were able to experience time away from their fears and anxieties about the future. In addition, being able to "do" and experience a sense of agency was something that participants found rewarding.'

When my daughters were born, all I wished for their future was health and happiness. Nothing seemed so vital to life except those two hopes; everything else could follow. Yet recently, they presented me with a fairy cake for my birthday, one candle pushed into it.

'Make a wish,' they said, and I blew it out and this time wished silently for health and happiness for myself.

But after they'd gone home, I looked around my living room and out of my window to the paddock beyond. Dusk was beginning to set in and the trees were bathed in an orange light. I felt happy, as I often do staring out at that scene. One out of two isn't bad, I thought to myself, thinking back to the wishes I had made. But then I never consider myself unhealthy, despite this disease inside my brain that makes it a little wonky and unreliable. I don't feel ill and I'm not in pain.

Perhaps the granting of those wishes is down to nothing except the perception of what those words mean to each and every one of us. I do face challenges every day, but perhaps mine are no greater than my neighbours'. We never really know what personal battle someone else is facing. So I had to ask myself whether those things I wished for were necessary after all, or if they had actually already been granted.

ATTITUDE

I'm staring out of the window of my bedroom, the room where I spend most time in daylight hours, and everything is the same: the tops of tall trees sway gently against a white midwinter sky and inside there is the gentle hum of my central heating. I am cosy and warm. Yet my head is a complete blank. I look down at my fingers moving across the keyboard, and then up at the words that appear on the screen. I read the words but feel no response stir inside. Somewhere, locked inside my body, I know that it is me who is making those words appear on the screen – it can be no one else – and yet they feel separate from me, as if I am looking over the shoulder of another person as they type. Perhaps, in some ways, I am.

These moments once felt like dramatic episodes that crashed into my brain like a tidal wave once every few weeks, rearranging all my thoughts and dragging others under. But now they occur so regularly – two or three times a week – that I have grown used to my life being disrupted like this. I know the signs now, yet the surge still overwhelms me, until it feels as if I am looking out at the world from under the mirrored surface of the water. It is close, everything looks the same, yet it is somehow unreachable for me.

I watch my fingers as they continue to move across the keyboard, the last piece of me still free from dementia, still living a life not dictated by this disease. What is their secret? How are they able to communicate with my brain? I wish I knew the answer, but instead I know not to question the respite that dementia has granted them – for now. Instead, while the rest of me is empty, they can express how I feel.

And then, just like that, those same fingers slow and tire before stopping altogether. The words no longer appear on the screen. I am alone.

I look around the room, telling myself that perhaps – like me – they just need time. I stare at the treetops again, encouraged that I can still remember that word for 'tree'. But there is something absent. I am not sure what. My mind scrambles to identify the missing link, but no thoughts come, not at first, nothing but this blankness. Until, yes, I realise – or some part of me does, because my fingers suddenly start typing again – and I see the missing word appear on the screen: 'smile'. I'm conscious then that my face is nondescript, that my lips make a straight line, that there is no indication to the outside world that I am here inside this moment. I am reduced to a shell of a person. If I were sitting in an armchair opposite, I know that's what anyone else would see.

What is missing is real emotion.

I cast a glance around the room, the buzzing, the short-circuiting inside my brain accompanying even the tiniest of movements. My eyes land on some photographs on the windowsill. That spark of recognition surfaces from the sludge of dementia. I know them well: there is my daughter Sarah; my other daughter, Gemma, on her wedding day to Stuart. Ordinarily, my eyes only have to fall on the sight of them for the emotion to well up inside, manifesting itself in a bright smile across my face – I feel it there. But now there is nothing. I'm aware of the skin and muscles of my face just hanging. These could be photographs of anyone. Is this how it will be? Is this my brain preparing me for the future, a future where I will not recognise the faces of the two people I love the most? I'd like to think then that Gemma and Sarah will be there to hold my hand, that the sense of touch, the sound of their voices will rouse me from this emptiness. That the emotion – that piece of me that makes me human – will still be summoned, stirred to the surface by the power of love.

But for now, I give in to the void. I put down my iPad and accept the haze and the blankness that it tucks me up in. I have a vague sense, somewhere in my bones, that the last time this happened – perhaps just a few days ago – the haze shifted when I did just this. When I gave in to dementia. Just for today, I sink under my duvet, and as I close my eyes, I glimpse those photographs on the windowsill again.

They will still be there when I wake, and hopefully, so will I...

ON THE BAD DAYS

I don't call them fogs any more, these moments when my brain short-circuits, when life becomes blurry and chaos reigns. It comes so often now that it feels better, somehow, to call them hazes. There is something about the word 'haze' that suggests something more temporary than fog, something that will be more certain to lift. The word suggests that I am there underneath all the time, just waiting for the mist to clear again. And it does.

That is another thing about these hazes: just like dementia itself, they have a beginning, a middle and an end. And after the end, there is the sunshine again, that crisp blue sky. The odd cloud still drifts by, but that is OK, I am still here.

It would make sense that these hazes come more frequently now. A sign perhaps of decline? After all, dementia is a progressive illness; there is no getting away from that. There was a time when I would have found this a frightening prospect, that my mind, in its clearer moments, would sense the end coming at me with more force. But I realise now that those thoughts only hasten me towards it. Better to keep it in perspective – that future isn't here yet, and it may be far, far away. How do any of us know for sure from one day to the next?

But in fact, the frequency of these hazes descending has brought with it a surprise. These moments of complete disorientation are bizarrely less frightening *because* of the frequency with which they arrive – and leave again. Because that is the important thing: not their arrival, but their departure. My brain keeps an imprint of that, a memory that they won't last, that they don't last. The frequency allows me to stay calm, to tell myself that it is nothing more that some faulty wiring inside my brain, a stray spark that has shut down the whole system, that this is perhaps my brain's way of coping. It is a physical action – or reaction – inside my body, but it is not me. And I always return to me. Yes, undoubtedly, a different me from the one before diagnosis. But how many of us can say we stay the same throughout our lives? The only difference with dementia is that these scars are more physical, more permanent, on the whole unmendable – yet not insurmountable.

But that all depends on how you look at things.

Attitude is half the battle when it comes to a disease like dementia. The way that we address these fogs, these short-circuits – call them what you like – can minimise or maximise what's happening to us. I asked some of my friends how they describe their less-good days:

'I describe them as my faint days. That most accurately reflects how I feel that day. It's not so much fog as faintness – fog feels too dramatic – instead it's a feeling that I'm just behind everything. It's like turning your head and then it all catches up a second later. You're just not quite there. For me, fog implies really you can't see anything – faintness is the closest I can get. I think a lot of my problems are to do with vascular dementia and oxygen literally not getting through to parts of my brain, so that word is also the most accurate when it comes to depicting the reality of those days. It minimises those episodes a little to describe them like that.'

'I get days where I can't think straight and make my breakfast – I'll end up putting salad cream on my muesli or blueberries in my coffee. That's when I might say my brain has gone off piste. I just laugh at the things I do, I know it's the dementia causing it, but I just laugh. I don't get down about it. If I do something silly when I'm out with my friends, I'll say, "Oh my brain's gone off-piste today," and they joke back: "Don't be playing that dementia card – it doesn't work with us." I just find humour helps me.'

'I describe those days as fuzzy days. I don't describe my Alzheimer's as Alzheimer's — I describe it as my sidekick, and I've done this right from the word go. I describe it as my sidekick because it's almost as if this person in my head comes and interferes with my daily routines and how I cope with things to cause me problems. So I always say it's my sidekick that's interfering with my day today. I describe my life now as a new chapter — my dementia chapter. On my bad days I don't know what I'm supposed to be doing, where I've been or what I've done. But on those days I just use my sidekick as my excuse. I think that makes it separate from me. It is separate because when I'm having my bad days it's like something that comes in and takes over my head, and leaves me slightly out of control, and I am a bit of a control freak, so this is why I have to have this other thing separate to me, my sidekick.'

ON DIAGNOSIS

The hardest thing for any human to cope with in life is a lack of control. Every one of us likes to go about our normal day-to-day business believing at least in the illusion that we are in control of our actions. For those of us living with dementia, this is the first thing that we are asked to accept — that we have an invader in our brains that has taken the wheel, that we are no longer at the controls. Except this isn't necessarily true. I have said many times already that dementia has a beginning, a middle and an end, and there is so much living to do if you — and those around you — can take a positive approach.

My 'foggy days' once appeared dramatic when they were new and disturbing, yet in some ways dementia has scored an own goal because their frequency now gives me back some control, some forewarning to set aside my diary for the day, or return back under the duvet.

This is my attitude today, six years into my diagnosis, and I realise that this is not the attitude of everyone who has received a devastating diagnosis of dementia. And there is no doubt that it is that: devastating. Certainly, at fifty-eight, when I sat across from a neurologist and was told that I had dementia, I didn't feel positive or in control. I heard the words that there was nothing more that they could do, and I left the hospital feeling that the end of my life had rushed to meet me. Who knew that six years later I would be writing my second book on the subject; that I would have spent the last few years travelling up and down the country to conferences and book festivals; that I would be giving talks to student nurses and experts in the field; that I would chat every day with people who like me had been blindsided by a diagnosis, giving them hope that far from it being the end, it might just be a different beginning. But for most of us who have been diagnosed, the most frightening prospect was that lack of control.

My friends have had a similar experience to me. The diagnosis that they were convinced in the beginning was the end of the world has instead opened up for them a different way of living – but living all the same:

'I've been diagnosed for eight years now, and when I got my diagnosis, it was very negative and I was afraid. I was led to believe from then on my life and future were structured and I tackled it. I was told to do what everybody else said, so I felt I'd lost myself. But eight years on, knowing what I know now and the friends I've met, my attitude has changed for the positive, because I know different now. I don't do as I'm told any more. I'll take advice on board and then I'll decide for myself. Seeing others living positively and my own experience, I still live my life positively. I don't think of the future; I live my life day by day.'

'I was diagnosed two years ago and I found the process very negative. I am quite a pessimistic person anyway – I've always looked at what could go wrong, and what might go wrong. Deep down I knew what it was, but I didn't want to admit it to myself. My dad kept saying: "There's nobody in the family who had dementia, so you'll be fine." But my grandma had dementia, and my granddad had Parkinson's disease. I was searching for information on Google and reading books, and some of that reading was so negative. I read a lot of books from the carer's point of view, and all of that was so negative, it was all about how they were struggling to cope with people, and all the time I was reading I had in my head: "This is how I'm going to be." When I got my diagnosis, I was gutted. But then I read your book *Somebody I Used to Know* and it totally changed my attitude. I thought: "If this lady could do it, then I can do it; nobody is going to stop me from doing what I'm doing now."'

ON COPING

Researchers from three British universities wanted to understand how set in stone people's attitudes were after diagnosis, and decided to visit them a year on to see how much had changed. Their 2005 report highlighted the fact that people's different coping mechanisms could be responsible for the ways outsiders perceive they are dealing with their disease. Some people, the report argues, cope with their diagnosis by denying it outwardly, yet this denial itself is often misinterpreted by others as a symptom of the disease itself. Coping styles are broken down into two modes: self-maintaining and self-adjusting. Those who fall into the category of self-maintaining might be the ones who do not acknowledge their dementia – for example, they might try to cover up or dismiss their forgetfulness, rather than implementing methods to aid them to cope better, as someone who is of the self-adjusting mindset might.

Neither is right or wrong, of course; we all cope as we see fit. But this lack of understanding about individual coping styles may lead family and friends to believe that the person living with dementia is not aware of this invader in their brains. 'In terms of social context,' the report's authors write.

> People with dementia who appear 'unaware' in one context may demonstrate very clear awareness in another. While this may reflect a genuinely fluctuating level of awareness, the variation may also arise because people adjust what they choose to express according to their preceptions of how it will be received or the impact it will have. Similarly, people with dementia who are said by those around them to be 'unaware' of their diagnosis or situation sometimes make it very clear in research

interviews that they are far more aware than has been assumed.

I have known people who will refuse to admit they have dementia, but are aware of the effects it's having on them. It's a strange mix. I liken it sometimes to people 'coming out' as gay – they know they are gay and are totally aware of it, but they fear the act of 'coming out'. Similar discriminations can exist for those of us with dementia, especially as some people still think of the disease as a mental illness and, sadly, we know there is a huge stigma undeservedly attached to that. It's no wonder that people might try to 'self-maintain' by minimising or dismissing their diagnosis when they don't feel safe to be themselves. But I've also known people who, for this reason, refuse to attend support groups with peers who could help to change their attitude about what it's like to live with dementia. When they're asked why, people respond: 'I just want to carry on living my life as normal and not think about dementia.' That is completely understandable, but their fear of acknowledging the disease may prevent them getting support from the very people who could really help. The only thing that would change their willingness to accept their own diagnosis would be if the attitude of society as a whole changed.

For most people interviewed by the author of the report, there was a change over the course of that year. I know I moved from grief to acceptance, which is what helps me to live as well as I can today. We constantly change and adapt, like humans do in any challenging situation. One coping mechanism doesn't necessarily stay with us throughout.

'In terms of individual psychological responses, the onset of dementia can be viewed as a threat to self that may trigger compensatory attempts at adaptive coping,' the report continues.

The coping style an individual adopts will be influenced by his or her personality and past experience, through which the individual has built up preferred ways of dealing with difficult situations. While some people cope by confronting difficulties head-on, many cope by attempting to minimise the threats they are experiencing. They may, for example, overtly seek to normalise or explain away any difficulties, or they may covertly avoid thinking about them, or there may be a more automatic or unconscious process of denying the difficulties.

Recognising someone's coping strategy is a vital step in helping them to live their best life with the disease. If for some that means not acknowledging it, then that's just the way they want to cope outwardly – but it doesn't mean that inside they are unaware of their dementia. People see me and my friends who are 'activists' in this area, and they perhaps don't want to live a life that appears consumed by the presence of dementia. Perhaps this is the right decision because our work can be all-consuming and that in some ways is a negative. Other people seem to be able to switch off, but some of us can't because of the fact that we have shared our stories publicly. But as the 2005 report says: 'There is a distinction to be made between unawareness and a conscious preference to avoid thinking or talking about possibly distressing issues, which might rather reflect a means of adaptive coping.'

Coping styles is an interesting area of research. A 2002 study found:

> Attempts at holding on and compensating were essentially self-protective, and reflected attempts to maintain a sense of self and normality. Developing a fighting spirit and coming to terms reflected attempts to confront the threats head-on, view them as a challenge, and respond in a way that balanced struggle with acceptance in order to integrate the changes within the self.

The important thing to remember is that no one coping strategy is the right one. The way we cope with adversity is as individual as we are – with or without dementia in tow.

ON THE ATTITUDES OF PROFESSIONALS

What many of us agree on is that it is the attitudes of the professionals that play the biggest part in how we feel about our own diagnosis. That is what I have learned most of all in these last six years: not only the power of my own attitude, but how that is influenced by those around me. That's why I prefer to be surrounded by positive people now – those who have a similar 'can do' attitude to me. But the only way this can filter down to others who are diagnosed is if the professionals take a different approach. Could the doctor who handed me my diagnosis have not put it in more positive terms? Could she not have said: 'Yes, this is a bummer of a disease, but this new label will not define you, you are still the same person who walked through this door five minutes ago – there is still so much you can do and be.' How differently I would have left her office then.

But six years on, not much has changed for me in terms of how I'm spoken to by professionals. It feels as if those of us with dementia have learned a lot more than doctors and nurses have. It is for this reason that I don't even attend my assessments any more: who wants to be told that they've deteriorated but there's nothing that can be done? It would be different if they voiced it in a different way, perhaps: 'It seems you're finding this area more challenging now, but let's see what we can put in place to help...' but they don't. And I am not the only one who feels this way among my peers:

'I no longer go for any assessments; they just make me feel negative. The last time I went they tested me to see if I'd deteriorated and they made a mistake because they went too far back in my medical history. They said I'd deteriorated quite a lot and were planning on changing my medication. I was a bit upset about it, wondering what the side effects of the new medication would be. Then I got a letter from them to say they were very sorry, but I was actually still on the same level – the lady had gone back too far to my previous assessments. I'd spent a month feeling really down and upset because of what they told me and it turned out it was wrong all the time, so I thought, I'm not going any more, so I don't get that kind of negativity in my life.'

'It's a feeling that the medical professionals are writing us off. They say: "There's nothing we can do and you just have to do what we tell you and prepare for the end.'''

'It's the professionals who can make you feel negative or positive about your diagnosis. A social worker phoned up a few months ago and asked if we could we make an appointment for her to come and have a chat with me. I live in a one-bedroom apartment; it's not sheltered housing, just an ordinary ground-floor flat, but I've got two friends living across the road. I know they are there, and my family are local, but the social worker came and said: "I've been thinking that it's time to go into sheltered housing." I said: "No, I get more care here than I would there." But because I live alone, she naturally assumed it was time for me to move to somewhere else to get looked after.'

'There's one GP I know, very experienced, who has said to me on more than one occasion: "Do you think they've got the diagnosis wrong? You can't have dementia." What she meant was "you can cook, you can talk – you can't have dementia". She says the usual things like, "Well, I keep losing my keys, or forgetting what I went into a room for." But she's sixty-five – you do at that age, but that's not dementia. Another thing the professionals do is they don't make allowances or adjustments for you; they know you have dementia but they still expect you to fill out the same forms and tell your story umpteen times. And if you go into hospital for an operation, they'll ask you on the morning of the operation: "Have you had anything to eat or drink?" What a stupid question; they shouldn't ask the question because they can't rely on the answer.'

'After I was diagnosed, I found the lack of support very disappointing. All the people at the memory clinic were saying things like, "Don't forget you've got to sort your will out," and, "Make sure you've got your life in order – you don't know how long you've got." The only medical professional for me who was positive was my own GP. I went back to see him because I didn't know whether to take the medication or not, and I was mulling it over and it was actually him who talked me through it, and in a way he helped me make my mind up not to take it. He said: "Just get out there and live your life, just do what you want to do." He was the only professional who said that to me.'

It is subjective, but how professionals make us feel can make us or break us. For so long professionals used negative words to describe us, simply because I think they didn't know how to react. It's only in the last few years that they've realised the negative effects these words have on patients. If you continually tell a child she's rubbish, in the end she'll start to believe it. Why wouldn't it be the same for adults? If we're continually referred to as challenging or disruptive, then it will affect us in the same way.

In her 2019 study, Emma Wolverson aimed to investigate the impact of language. In a survey of 378 health and social care professionals, none could agree on which term they preferred to describe those with dementia. What they did agree on, though, was that 'words are very powerful and the professionals who took part in our study felt the words used to describe changes in behaviours would influence how other people responded to and tried to help the person with dementia'. Disrepecful and offensive language more often than not leads to substandard care.

People with dementia agreed that they did not like terms like 'challenging behaviour' and liked instead terms like 'unmet needs'. 'People preferred terms that were kind and didn't make them feel daft or guilty. There were some very strong reactions by some people who were worried that the wrong label would lead to poor care and the person with dementia no longer being treated like a person.'

I can understand how that would be a frightening prospect, especially in a care home where you are so reliant on others for care. None of us wants dementia to define who we are – we want to hold on to our self, just as someone with cancer isn't defined by the cancer. But those of us living with dementia seem to be labelled more easily, and assumptions are made because of that label. How we behave when communication is difficult often isn't our fault. If someone is giving you coffee when you only drink tea and the only way of showing that dislike is by throwing the cup on the floor, that's the only way. But that is indicative of an unmet need, not difficult or challenging behaviour.

Wolverson's report concluded: 'In this study people with dementia shared significant concerns that some of the language regularly used by health and social care professionals placed people with dementia at serious risk of harm because they are seen as symptoms to be treated rather than seeing the whole person.'

This makes me feel very sad. It is so important for the professionals who are caring for us to have the right attitude, and this shows through the language they use. If they can't get it right, they are simply not qualified for the job.

ON THE ATTITUDES OF FAMILY

The good news is that every new day offers us a chance to start again, to change the language we use, the tone, the way we approach a progressive disease – whether you are the one diagnosed yourself, or perhaps, even more importantly, if you are someone who supports a person who is, be that in the family, the community or the medical profession. It is never too late to make a change. You can start the moment you put this book down.

Our attitudes when it comes to dealing with traumatic events in life can change. Think about things that have happened in your own life: deaths, divorce, redundancy. People undoubtedly go through a period of mourning, of readjustment, but in the end they reach acceptance and look for the best that life has to offer – so why should dementia be any different?

My attitude is simply my way of coping. It is no better, or worse, than anybody else's. I am able to turn these ever-increasing hazes into a positive because I'm lucky enough to feel them coming. Some of my friends have no signs that their particular haze is coming, or perhaps they don't read the signs, or choose not to. I'm lucky that I have an instinctive nature that questions how my head feels on any given day, but others aren't so fortunate. It doesn't mean they've failed somehow. I cope with my dementia by 'doing'. It is not the same for everyone.

We each have our own individual tactic for facing life and this disease, but when those around us disable us, it changes the way we go about our life. I asked my friends how their family had reacted to their diagnoses:

'For me the reaction from my friends and family was very negative, which brings you down, they are not positive about it, and it is still classed by some people as an old person's disease. At the beginning I was taking in all this negativity and I was trying my best to say to people, "I'm going to be OK," but deep down I was thinking: "Am I going to be OK?"'

'My brother is a year older than me and he's never accepted my diagnosis. I don't know whether it's fear that he might get it. I've tried to explain it to him, but he doesn't understand and he doesn't want to understand. My mum passed away about fourteen years ago now, but a couple of years ago I'd gone out with my brother one lunchtime to the social club, and when it was time to leave I said to him: "I've got to wait, Mum's going to meet me here." He said: "No, Mum's dead." And I said: "No, she's meeting me here." Of course, I know my mum's dead, but at that moment, I must have been confused. He shouted at me, he dragged me across the car park, I was hanging on to a lamp post saying: "Mum's coming – I've got to wait here." He was shouting and dragging me and everyone came out of the social club to see what was going on. One woman phoned an ambulance saying: "We've got a lady here with dementia."'

'The next day my brother came round to mine and I apologised to him. My daughter went mad when

I told her. She said: "Why did you say you're sorry? He should have been the one to say sorry." She's right that he caused that distress because he was trying to take me into reality and at that moment my reality was that I needed to stay and wait for Mum. If he had listened to me when I had been trying to explain what dementia's like, he wouldn't have acted that way, but he doesn't want to listen. My daughter said don't go out with him again on your own because if anything like that happens again, he would react wrongly. It would have been better in that situation if he'd said: "We'll sit here for a while, but Mum did ring me and say she might not make it today." I was just so upset and very emotional after that incident. I didn't go to that social club for ages afterwards because I was embarrassed because all those people had come out to see what was going on and they probably thought I'd had too much to drink.'

It's true that in the first case, my friend's apology was for her brother's ignorance, and she's right that if only he had tried to understand what it felt like to have dementia inside your brain, he would have been able to handle the situation better for both of them. Instead his reaction left her feeling upset and embarrassed.

As one friend said to me:

'We spend a lot of time understanding that others don't understand our dementia, and how we are and how we feel. We end up having to make allowances for them. We often have to accommodate others' lack of insight and empathy, and to do that we have to disown our own feelings. We have to deny the reality of what's going on in our heads – in terms of our feelings – just because other people don't understand. But it makes us feel worse because we can't be ourselves. It's a curious mix. We want to be nice to other people and accept that they don't have the insight or understanding of dementia, but by doing that we're denying our own feelings.'

This is why education is important. People can't be expected to know what they don't know and that even includes those who are our nearest and dearest. But they have come to these conclusions about dementia because of what they've seen or heard in society, and perhaps also because of what they've refused to see or hear because they're scared of a disease like dementia.

The attitude of others will influence how the person living with dementia feels about themselves, and therefore how well they cope with their diagnosis. A 2004 study looked at how complex the behaviour can be of someone living with dementia: 'A person who insists to the clinic that all is well may do so out of a fear of being "put away", or a sense that forgetfulness is minor compared to other health problems, or a need to maintain self-esteem,' the report said.

The same person may, in the family setting, express fear and distress about what is happening, or show this indirectly through his or her behaviour. Partners' accounts indicate that they are often highly attuned to underlying meanings, seeking to support coping strategies in an attempt to reinforce a person's sense of self. Clinicians, too, need to be sensitive to the psychological needs of the person with Alzheimer's as demonstrated in the way in which they describe their subjective experience, and must be ready to respond in a way that enhances well-being.

Here's a different scenario that another friend told me about:

'My parents are in their eighties and I'm an only child as well, which made it even worse telling them that I'd been diagnosed with young-onset dementia at fifty-four. It was a bigger shock for them than it was for me. My mum couldn't talk to me, which I found so difficult, especially when I was still processing the diagnosis myself. On top of that, not to have your parents to be able to speak to you about how you're feeling about it was very difficult. My mum asked me straight away: "How long have you got to live?" At the time that was very hurtful but as I've thought about it further, I've put myself in her position and wondered how I would have felt if that was my daughter. I'd have given her a hug, I know that, which my mum and dad didn't do. I didn't get a hug; it was like I'd been pushed away. My dad saw it as a flaw in the family history. My dad, being a perfectionist, was asking where had this disease come from. It really affected him. It took some getting over for me to come to terms with the fact that my mum and dad couldn't accept it. Now my mum sort of gets it — she rings me and messages me. She doesn't exactly say she's proud of me — she never has

done; she finds it really hard to say things like that —
but I know deep down that they are proud of me, but
it's the fact that they haven't said it. But now my uncle
has just been diagnosed and Mum said: "He's living in
that house on his own and they're not putting him into
a home." And I said: "Well, he won't want to go into a
home. They might have asked him what he wants." And
she said: "How's he going to cope on his own?" And
I said: "Well, he will, most probably better in his own
home, because he's in familiar surroundings, he knows
that place, he knows where things are." But even now,
my mum still thinks everyone with dementia should go
into a home.'

My friend's experience of having to reveal her own
diagnosis to her elderly parents is a scenario that until
the writing of this book I had not considered before. It
was a shame that due to their own prejudices about what
dementia meant to their family, they weren't able to offer
their daughter the comfort that she needed from her mum
and dad in that moment — our parents are always our
parents, whatever age we are. It had never occurred to
me that with more people being diagnosed with young-
onset dementia — representing around 5 per cent of all
those diagnosed — this could be a situation that becomes
increasingly common within families. But if we don't
talk about dementia, if we don't educate people, how are
attitudes meant to change? It is true that it often ends up
being the person with dementia who does the comprom-
ising, who hides their feelings so as not to upset someone,
but if we can't speak up about situations and scenarios we

find challenging, then we just end up disabling ourselves
further.

ON A SENSE OF SELF

The idea of self, and the importance of hanging on to it,
has been well-documented in dementia research. Once
that sense of self starts to slip, alongside autobiographical
memories, the decline seems to get steeper. Memories
make us who we are, but they also enable those who didn't
know us historically to see us as a whole person, to understand our needs and our actions. We mustn't lose sight of
our past because it makes us what we are in the future.

We often lose our sense of self when diagnosed. We
feel we are not of value any more, perhaps a bit like when
people retire and feel that they have lost that sense of purpose. In Marie Mills's 1997 study, one man with advanced
dementia was able to talk in great detail about his time as a
prisoner of war. Researchers noted the importance of this:

> They were the type of memories which ... 'live long in
> the memory of the mind,' for they tended to be signifi-
> cantly concerned with the individual physical and psy-
> chological survival of the self. The intensity of effort to
> survive during his time as a prisoner of war may have
> created these durable memories which appeared to
> withstand the onslaught of dementia, almost until the
> end ... His stories allowed him to be readily seen as a
> 'whole' person. This gave him a sense of narrative iden-
> tity and underlines the importance of the maintenance
> of narrative during this illness.

All of us want to be seen as more than just dementia. It fosters for both us and others a better attitude towards the disease. I have spoken in these pages about how much I liked being known as Wendy the 'camera lady' in my village, instead of Wendy with dementia. It was refreshing for me because people saw my skills before they saw my dementia – they saw the person rather than the disease.

There will come a time when we are not capable of sharing stories about the person we were before dementia, and that's why we always say that the people closest to us know us best and should be listened to. They are the keepers of our history when communication becomes difficult, but these stories of ours can also be shared with other carers as a way of connecting and making relationships with them. If these stories are shared, they can then be returned to us, and they might explain our actions better. It brings to mind an anecdote I heard of an ex-nurse who used to sit behind the nurses' station in her care home. The care assistants didn't know why she would get so cross if they tried to make her go to her room. Once they learned she used to be a nurse herself, they allowed her to sit there and shuffle papers and write pretend notes. Or the man who used to be a milkman who was labelled as 'disruptive' because he got up at 4 a.m. every day and went in search of milk bottles in the kitchen to place outside residents' rooms. He used to get angry and violent when they tried to stop him – wouldn't you, if someone was interfering with your job? – but once they found out he used to be a milkman, they allowed him to deliver milk in the early hours. When he'd finished and gone 'home' to bed, staff would remove them before everyone else woke up.

This sharing of autobiographical detail should be vital to any care plan, as the Mills report confirmed:

> As informants became more cognitively impaired by their disease there was an awareness ... that they had bequeathed their narrative to another. It is argued that the sharing of such a narrative, within dementia care, reinforces carer attitudes of respect, understanding and acceptance. In this sense, therefore, the personal narrative ... is never lost. It continues its existence in the form of a valuable resource which can be returned to them, either verbally or non-verbally, during subsequent interactions. Thus, care plans and all care approaches and conversations will be influenced by carer knowledge and understanding of the client. This should continue throughout the process of dementia, even during the latter stages, when the ability to communicate with others is severely compromised.

ON POSITIVITY

A 2020 study by Hannah Scott looked into women's attitudes towards their dementia. It concluded that those around us have a huge impact on how women see themselves after a diagnosis, and that the more they were able to maintain a social life, the more positive attributes were reflected back to them, thus boosting their self-esteem as well as their self-concept.

The report discussed how women's determination to enrich their lives with a wide range of activities brought them 'happiness and a sense of purpose'. 'Maintaining their independence was also important to many women, which was expressed by a desire to have control over decisions and aspects of their life. This was achieved through coping strategies – the use of diaries and calendars, for example, were particularly important to those women living alone.'

The study affirmed that 'maintaining a positive self-concept was central to the overall theme of resistance. This allowed people to perceive themselves in a positive light, reinforcing capabilities and thereby protecting self-esteem.'

I can see why these coping strategies lead to more positivity for women, but there is no reason why they shouldn't apply to men too. I have always talked of the importance of not giving up on ourselves – so many others will try to do that for us – and it is essential to keep a positive attitude, to focus on what we can still do, activities we can still involve ourselves in, and finding solutions – like the diaries and calendars mentioned here – to make them happen. All of this leads to a more positive attitude.

The report also talked about the negativity that women faced from family members, and how that differed from their own attitude: 'Women were hopeful that deterioration was not an inevitability and that they could continue as they were. Family members, on the other hand, believed that uncertainty was a reason to be fearful of the future, and the inability to know "how bad" dementia would get.'

I asked my friends about whether their own friends and family had been able to instil in them a positive outlook:

'My family's attitude has changed since they've seen me being positive and taking these positive risks. They've been more positive about it because they're seeing that it's not the end for me, I'm not going to become that burden. My son said the other day that he's so proud of me. He was the one who was more negative about the diagnosis. He didn't like me going off travelling on trains – he thought I should be at home because I was ill – but only yesterday he said: "I'm really proud of you, Mum. The way you're getting on with things, and keeping your independence." Life is a risk from the day you're born, but I'm not going to let dementia define me, and my family have learned that if they don't allow me to do the things that I did before dementia, then it will take over.'

'My husband has been brilliant. He just lets me carry on with whatever I want to do and he never ever says to me, "You can't do that," which is absolutely brilliant. Sometimes I just wish he would take over when I'm having one of the bad days, but for me, I always fight through those bad days. I never rest, I'm always on the go, but my hubby just lets me do anything, he's letting me do the things I want to do, which I'm very grateful for, because I've seen people in groups where the husband or the wife takes over and won't let people do anything for themselves – won't even let them speak – but we need to carry on doing what we're doing.'

'As soon as you mention you have Alzheimer's disease, the reaction you get from people is really negative. But now if we meet anybody and they say: "Oh, I haven't seen you for ages," and you get talking and say: "I got a diagnosis of Alzheimer's," and they gasp and I stop them right there and say: "Oh no, don't be sorry – I'm enjoying myself." Because I think I am having a good life at the moment, I'm doing what I want to do and what I like to do.'

ON PEER SUPPORT

I still remember that first time attending Minds and Voices in York, a local support group for those living with dementia. The hesitancy about actually going. I wasn't, after all, a 'group person'. I never had been. But something drew me towards this one: the need to see and hear others in the same situation as me, and to know I was not alone. I had attended a WOW (Women of the World) conference and heard Agnes Houston speak about the power of peer support, and so, tentatively, I went along.

Most of all, I can still conjure up that feeling of calmness, of relaxing into my seat, finally feeling as though I was among friends, among people who understood and wouldn't judge me in the same way I wouldn't judge them in return. We could just 'be'.

Six years on, I still get the same feeling when I enter a room where my friends are sitting. So many friendships have blossomed since those early connections with Minds and Voices. We greet each other now like long-lost friends and call each other our second family. George calls me 'sister', and I call him 'my bro', such is the closeness that we feel.

My friends and I would never have met if dementia hadn't crossed our paths. Many of us have had to accept that our old, familiar friendships have disappeared. We know so little about one another's pasts – we probably wouldn't remember the detail anyway – but we share a diagnosis of dementia and that is enough to create an instant bond.

Meeting other people with dementia was what changed my attitude towards the disease, and I asked my friends what it had meant to them:

> 'Among my peers, we are a very tiny percentage of the people who have a diagnosis, or indeed live without a diagnosis of dementia, and there are so many people out there I imagine who never get near our positivity, our attitude, because they never meet us, they never meet other people. They maybe have family or spouses who are very negative about it all. I have heard stories about people who are not allowed out of the house because their wife or husband doesn't want people to see them. I have heard stories about people who say their friends have stopped visiting them because they want to remember them how they were, not how they are now. There is so much support out there, and so many people never get this invaluable experience of meeting peers.'

> 'I felt alone after my diagnosis; there were no groups that I knew about – I didn't even know where to turn to. I found the lady from the Alzheimer's Society very patronising – she was talking to me like a child: "Ooh you're doing well, you're looking lovely today." That wasn't what I needed – I needed some direction of where I was going. Finding the local group was a bit of a turning point. There was a man there who was coping well with his diagnosis and he'd been diagnosed quite some time before. I suppose when I entered that group

for the first time, it was very scary because I didn't know what I was going to find, and I didn't know what these people were going to be like because I'd never met anyone with dementia of my age. But there were people who were a lot older and there were people who were my age and, suddenly, I didn't feel so alone.'

'I've found all these people who are doing things and supporting one another and talking to each other and this is how we educate ourselves. For me my turning point was meeting everybody and everybody was so positive. We don't think about negative things now.'

'It's how other people interact with you that can change how you feel about your diagnosis. Before you meet other peers, there's a sense that you are alone in a world of everything else being normal and you are not. I know a lot of people feel intensely dark and lost and probably suicidal at times for the first few months after the diagnosis, and some never come out of that. But meeting other people and forming those new friendship groups, that is what makes life zing again. We are who we are; we're not odd; we're not written off.'

'There's the professionals again giving you all this negativity and it's people living with dementia who give you positivity. I'm more for positive risk taking; if I die, then I'll die happy.'

The Scott study also talked of the benefits of support groups: 'The literature on support groups for people with dementia has found that they have the potential to improve depressive symptoms and quality of life and increase self-esteem. They provide opportunities for participants to showcase their retained capabilities and to express their fears and emotions in a supportive environment.'

Obviously all groups will be different, so sometimes it's a case of finding the right one for you. But the report found that 'enabling and encouraging participation in such groups could enhance selfhood and by implication well-being. This connects to the wider issue of decreasing the stigma of dementia, to the point that people living with the disease do not attempt to engage in the tiring process of modifying or hiding their symptoms, for fear of societal rejection.'

In an ideal world, there wouldn't be any need for these niche groups. We only really have peer support groups because society won't make the adjustments that would allow us to integrate. Why should we have to create a separate art group for people with dementia when an ordinary art group would be just as satisfying? I remember the choir I joined and how much I loved being a part of it, but I had to leave because the organiser refused to allow me to hold a piece of paper on stage so I could read the words to the songs.

Maybe in the future we'll be able to openly talk to anyone about our diagnoses, but until we reach this utopia, peer support offers the safest, most relaxed and non-judgemental environment for any of us. And usually, a good laugh as well.

We understand, we trust, we don't judge, we share, we care and we're there to support one another through whatever dementia throws at us. Maybe we could teach the world a very simple lesson that acceptance and understanding of others is possible, and if those of us with a complex brain disease know that, it can't be too difficult for everyone else.

EPILOGUE

I'm sitting in front of my GP with a piece of paper in my hand that I need her signature on.

'I've got a little favour to ask,' I say.

She looks back, puzzled.

'I need your permission for something.'

I push the piece of paper across the desk to her, and as she opens it, I see her forehead crease with confusion.

'You're going to do a skydive?' she says finally.

A few months later, I wake and very soon there is a smile on my face. I hold my breath, listen out for the wind rattling at my window, any warning sign that today's flight won't be able to take place, like so many days before this one. But all I can hear are the birds. It's a good sign, especially as today I would be heading skywards to join them.

It has been months now since I saw the advert by Young Dementia UK, a charity I'm always involved with in some way. This year they wanted to raise funds by organising skydives. Perhaps they had expected relatives or carers to offer to take part. But I was fit and well, and who says people with dementia can't jump out of planes?

We drive along under a blue sky. I had wondered whether my GP would agree to sign the medical waiver. I knew that unless she said yes, the organiser wouldn't allow it. But luckily for me, since she read my first book she has changed her view about dementia. And so it was that when I asked her, she rolled her eyes, shook her head, and with a smile curling at her lips, she signed the paper.

As Gemma and I see signs to the airfield, I remember the last time I headed here for the flight I took in a glider. The pilot had taken my daughters to one side before the flight and asked if I was up to it. I tried not to take offence, knowing that attitude of disbelief was just another reason why I needed to write a book about the subject. And so I did – once I came back down to earth, of course.

As we get closer to the turn-off, traffic starts to back up. I glance at the sat nav, which says we'll be there in ten minutes, but I wonder if it has accounted for all of these cars. Gemma must sense my anxiety, my fear of being late to anywhere.

'You're getting stressed about a queue of traffic but you're not worried about jumping out of a plane?' she laughs.

Whenever I have spoken to people about this latest madcap plan of mine, there has always been a pause, disbelief collected in their eyes. I feel then the need to lighten the situation and put their minds at rest, reminding them that I would be jumping out of a plane at 10,000 feet strapped to someone else – there was no fear I would forget to open my own parachute.

'So I can just relax and enjoy myself,' I shrugged.

I'm not sure they were convinced.

I wonder why there is so much risk aversion. Dementia or not, my quality of life is as important as the next person's, and I want mine to be filled with experience and adventure. Why wouldn't I?

As I sit beside Gemma, laughing at my fear of tardiness but not of freefalling, I know there is no way she would consider jumping out of a plane. But her positive, supportive attitude means I can do so without worry. Both my daughters have always enabled me, providing constant encouragement despite their own initial shock and horror of whatever it is I want to do next. They've let go of worry in the same way I have. They just allow me to enjoy, and for that, I am forever grateful.

We finally pull off the main road and into the airfield. There I am introduced to my fellow skydivers and all the paperwork I am required to fill in. No one mentions dementia, not even as we sit with a cuppa watching all the other parachutes descend from the clouds.

Finally, my name is called. One final hug for Gemma and I head off for training. It is, of course, utterly hilarious for me. My instructor gives us lots of instructions, often accompanied by a long list of 'musts' and an even longer one of 'must nots'. I capture one – you must lift your feet when landing. That'll have to do.

I make jokes to put the others at ease – particularly the woman who has been 'surprised' by her family that morning with a skydive for her fiftieth birthday.

I stand beside a young woman who is also doing her jump for charity. The two guys who will be filming us make polite conversation. I mention then that I'm jumping for Young Dementia UK.

'Because I have dementia,' I tell them.

They take it in, but don't bat an eyelid – after all, these are people of the same mindset as me; those who love jumping out of aeroplanes for kicks, the ones who crave adventure. I know they won't consider me a liability.

My jumpsuit is placed in front of me, but I stare down, not knowing which arm or leg to put where. Suddenly, a giant of a man, all dressed in pink, strides towards me.

'Come on, let me help you get into this contraption,' he says calmly, his voice not fitting his stature somehow. 'We're going to make this a day to remember.'

I don't like to say anything to him.

From then on, I call him Mr Pink Man, and I have no fear, just complete confidence that he will see me up into the sky and safely back down to earth. All eyes are on me as I prepare to walk over to the plane. Onlookers have gathered around Gemma, their eyes darting to and from me with concern, as if saying: 'Should she be doing this?'

I give her one last hug, and just for extra reassurance tell her: 'I'm so excited!'

The red-and-blue jumpsuit I'm wearing is so cumbersome that I waddle towards the plane. It takes two men to hoist me in. I'm surprised to see the inside is an empty shell, no seats, just the floor to sit on. The other people join us, and before long we are rumbling along the airstrip. As we start our ascent, the plane's engines roar in my ears. I distract myself with the stunning views over the coastline as Mr Pink Man gives me a running commentary of what we can see from up here – north through Filey, Flamborough Head, Scarborough and beyond to Robin Hood's Bay, and as the plane pitches south to gain height, my beloved Humber Bridge comes into sight.

The ascent to 10,000 feet takes around twenty minutes and a beeping signals that we've reached the right time to leap. Mr Pink Man fastens us tight together and we shuffle towards the open door of the plane.

'Head back, head back,' he repeats in my ear as the rush of cold air hits me, stealing my breath away.

And then we jump.

I am floating, the earth below me, Mr Pink Man strapped to my back like a turtle shell. We are higher than the birds.

We fall... faster... lower... 130 miles an hour fast, to be precise. We are freefalling down to earth and I am smiling, wider than I have ever smiled before. If this is not freedom, then I don't know what is. Up here, there is no dementia. Up here, that disease does not inhabit my brain. I am flying, free from all that binds me to the earth.

The jolt of the pink parachute takes me by surprise, and as it opens above us, so too does the peace, the silence, a sense of stillness as we float gently down towards earth. The clouds are our company, the ground a finished jigsaw.

A voice in my ear says: 'Do you fancy doing some acrobats and twirls?'

I hear myself replying: 'Yes!'

We whoosh through the air, spinning this way and that. I close my eyes at first, a sensation that my eyeballs might just vacate their sockets, but once I've adjusted, I peer out again and squeal with delight as the world whizzes by.

We right ourselves again. Up here it feels as if we're descending back down to earth so slowly, yet as the ground comes closer – and I spot Gemma waving, a tiny dot – I see we are actually travelling at an alarming rate.

'Legs up,' Mr Pink Man shouts in my ears as we come closer every second to the viewing area. I'm confused because I thought the landing spot was behind the woods.

'Legs up,' he says again.

But I am exhausted, from the thrill of it more than anything. I feel the smile still plastered to my face, as if the wind has left it there, but there is no energy left in me. Then I hear people shouting from the ground.

'Legs up, Wendy!'

Mr Pink Man must realise this and he lands us both like ducks on water, and I collapse in a heap at his feet.

'Did we miss the landing spot because of me?' I ask.

'No,' he says. 'We had to show everyone you could do it.'

He hugs me and undoes all the clips and fasteners. Two other men come and help me stagger back to the hangar to the sound of claps and cheers, and there I take off my jumpsuit.

I wrap Gemma in a huge hug and then a man from the crowd interrupts us. He takes a £20 note out of his wallet because he knows I'm doing this for charity.

'Amazing, well done,' he says, handing it to me.

Had he been one of the doubters as I took to the air? Who knows? In that moment I hardly care.

If I listened to what everyone else says, I would never have jumped out of an aeroplane. I would never have done half the things that others say are not possible for people living with dementia.

For now, back on terra firma, I'm still buzzing – and plotting my next adventure. Why on earth should they ever stop?

BIBLIOGRAPHY

SENSES

Collins, Lindsey, *Understanding the Eating and Drinking Experiences of People Living with Dementia and Dysphagia in Care Homes: A qualitative study of the multiple perspectives of the person, their family, care home staff and Speech and Language Therapists* (PhD thesis), University of Bradford, 2020

Morgan-Jones, Peter, Maggie Beer, Emily Colombage, Danielle McIntosh and Prudence Ellis, *Don't Give Me Eggs That Bounce: 118 Cracking Recipes for People with Alzheimer's*, HammondCare Media, 2014

Morgan-Jones, Peter, Lisa Greedy, Prudence Ellis and Danielle McIntosh, *It's All About the Food Not the Fork: 107 Easy to Eat Meals in a Mouthful*, HammondCare Media, 2016

Morgan-Jones, Peter, Rod MacLeod, Prudence Ellis and Jessica Lynch, *Lobster for Josino: Fabulous Food for Our Final Days*, HammondCare Media, 2018

Hanaoka, Hideaki, et al., 'Effects of Olfactory Stimulation On Reminiscence Practice in Community-Dwelling Elderly Individuals', *Psychogeriatrics*, vol. 18, issue 4, 26 July 2018, pp. 283–91

Glachet, Ophélie, et al., 'Smell Your Memories: Positive Effect of Odour Exposure on Recent and Remote Autobiographical Memories in Alzheimer's Disease', *Journal of Clinical and Experimental Neuropsychology*, 41 (6), August 2019, pp. 555–64

Glachet, Ophélie, et al., 'Smell Your Self: Olfactory Stimulation Improves Self-Concept in Alzheimer's Disease', *Neuropsychological Rehabilitation*, 20 October 2020

Moyle, Wendy, 'Exploring the Effect of Foot Massage on Agitated Behaviours in Older People With Dementia: A Pilot Study', *Australasian Journal on Ageing*, vol. 30, issue 3, 26 April 2011, pp. 159–61

RELATIONSHIPS

Parveen, Sahdia, et al., 'Involving minority ethnic communities and diverse experts by experience in dementia research: The Caregiving HOPE Study', *Dementia* (London), November 2018, 17 (8), pp. 990–1000

Odzakovic, Elzana, et al., *'It's Our Pleasure, We Count Cars Here': An exploration of the 'neighbourhood-based connections' for people living alone with dementia*, Cambridge University Press, 2019

COMMUNICATION

Gerritsen, D. et al., 'Ethical Implications of the Perception and Portrayal of Dementia', *Dementia* (London), July 2018, 17 (5), pp. 596–608. First published 2016

Talbot, Catherine V., et al., 'How People With Dementia Use Twitter: A Qualitative Analysis', *Computers in Human Behaviour*, vol. 102, January 2020, pp. 112–19

ENVIRONMENT

Odzakovic, Elzana, et al., '"Overjoyed That I Can Go Outside": Using walking interviews to learn about the lived experience and meaning of neighbourhood for people living with dementia', *Dementia*, vol. 19, 12 December 2018, pp. 2199–2219

Global Age-Friendly Cities: A Guide, World Health Organization, 2007

Dementia Friendly Communities: Global Developments, Alzheimer's Disease International, second edition, 2017

Easton, Tiffany and Julie Ratcliffe, 'The Economics of Design' in *Design, Dignity, Dementia: Dementia-related design and the built environment*, World Alzheimer Report, vol. 1, Alzheimer's Disease International, 2020

Quirke, Martin, et al., 'Citizen Audits: Developing a participatory, place-based approach to dementia-enabling neighbourhoods' in *Design, Dignity, Dementia: Dementia-related design and the built environment*, World Alzheimer Report, vol. 1, Alzheimer's Disease International, 2020

Odzakovic, Elzana, et al., *'It's Our Pleasure, We Count Cars Here': an exploration of the 'neighbourhood-based connections' for people living alone with dementia*, Cambridge University Press, 2019

Osborne, Ash, 'Home Modifications to Support People Living with Dementia' in *Design, Dignity, Dementia: Dementia-related design and the built environment*, World Alzheimer Report, vol. 1, Alzheimer's Disease International, 2020

Harrison, Stephanie, and Richard Fleming, in *Design, Dignity, Dementia: Dementia-related design and the built environment*, World Alzheimer Report, vol. 1, Alzheimer's Disease International, 2020

EMOTIONS

Mills, Marie, *Narrative Identity and Dementia: A Study of Emotion and Narrative in Older People with Dementia*, Cambridge University Press, 1997

Berry, Charlotte, *Exploring the Experience of Living with Young Onset Dementia* (doctoral thesis), University of Leeds, 2017

Kessler, Eva-Marie, et al., 'Dementia Worry: A Psychological Examination of an Unexplored Phenomenon', *European Journal of Ageing*, 9 (4), 22 September 2012, pp. 275–84

ATTITUDE

Clare, Linda, et al., 'Perceptions of Change Over Time in Early-Stage Alzheimer's Disease', *Dementia*, vol. 4, issue 4, 2005, pp. 487–520

Clare, Linda, 'We'll Fight it as Long as We Can: Coping with the Onset of Alzheimer's Disease', *Aging & Mental Health*, 6 (2), May 2002, pp. 139–48

Wolverson, Emma, et al., 'Naming and Framing the Behavioural and Psychological Symptoms of Dementia', *OBM Geriatrics*, vol. 3, issue 4, 2019

Clare, Linda, 'Managing Threats to Self: Awareness of Early Stage Alzheimer's Disease', *Social Science & Medicine*, 57 (6), September 2003, pp. 1017–29

Mills, Marie, *Narrative Identity and Dementia: A Study of Emotion and Narrative in Older People with Dementia*, Cambridge University Press, 1997

Scott, Hannah, *The Impact of Dementia on the Selfhood and Identity of Women: A Social Constructionist Approach*, Cardiff University, 2020

ACKNOWLEDGEMENTS

Despondency and self-doubt are easy bedfellows when you're diagnosed with dementia, but my book shows that you must never give up on yourself; others will do that for you.

But in this, my second book – who would have thought seven years ago that I would be typing those words? – I have so many people to be thankful to, for their support and encouragement.

My lovely collaborator and now friend, Anna Wharton, who despite having taken me on once with my first book decided it was fun enough to work with me again.

Thank you to Robert Caskie for supporting us so well. Huge thanks of course must go to Alexis Kirschbaum for having the belief in me for a second time, along with all the wonderful staff at Bloomsbury Publishing, including Jasmine Horsey, Sarah Ruddick, Kate Quarry, Stephanie Rathbone, Jonny Coward and Akua Boateng. With special thanks to David Mann, who once again came up with the perfect cover.

Thanks to all those researchers we mention in the book, who have decided on a career to help find the best ways to live with dementia, the best ways to care and the best ways to care for those unable to care for themselves. A special HUGE thanks to Professor Jan Oyebode, who tolerated my countless emails asking for help with patience and humour, along with my good friend Professor Pat Sikes and Dr Julie Christie for their constant help and support.

To all my friends living with dementia – particularly my three amigos, Gail, George and Dory, without whom this book simply couldn't have been written. You are all my stars, along with Innovations in Dementia, whose work enables us to demonstrate to the world at large that we CAN. I can't thank you all enough.

But my final thanks must go to five others this time around. To the most important people in my life: Sarah, Gemma and Stuart. Without their understanding, love and continued willingness to travel this life with me, I would be in a very different, lonely place. And to Billy and Merlin, who provide the furry cuddles and unconditional love and laughter.

Please feel free to read my blog following my countless escapades: www.whichmeamitoday.wordpress.com

Or follow me on Twitter: @WendyPMitchell

A NOTE ON THE AUTHOR

Wendy Mitchell spent twenty years as a non-clinical team leader in the NHS before being diagnosed with young-onset dementia in July 2014 at the age of fifty-eight. Shocked by the lack of awareness about the disease, both in the community and in hospitals, she vowed to spend her time raising awareness about dementia and encouraging others to see that there is life after a diagnosis. In 2019 she was awarded an honorary Doctor of Health by the University of Bradford for her contribution to research. She has two daughters and lives in Yorkshire.

A NOTE ON THE TYPE

The text of this book is set in Perpetua. This typeface is an adaptation of a style of letter that had been popularised for monumental work in stone by Eric Gill. Large scale drawings by Gill were given to Charles Malin, a Parisian punch-cutter, and his hand-cut punches were the basis for the font issued by Monotype. First used in a private translation called 'The Passion of Perpetua and Felicity', the italic was originally called Felicity.